Medical Management of Psychotropic Side Effects

Aniyizhai Annamalai

Medical Management
of Psychotropic Side Effects

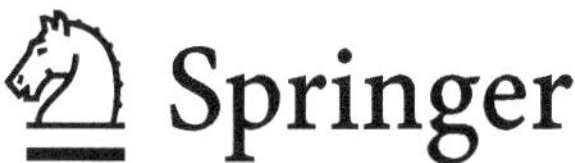 Springer

Aniyizhai Annamalai, MD
Departments of Internal Medicine & Psychiatry
Yale University School of Medicine
New Haven, CT, USA

ISBN 978-3-319-51024-8   ISBN 978-3-319-51026-2   (eBook)
DOI 10.1007/978-3-319-51026-2

Library of Congress Control Number: 2016961208

Printed on acid-free paper

This Springer imprint is published by Springer Nature
The registered company is Springer International Publishing AG
The registered company address is: Gewerbestrasse 11, 6330 Cham, Switzerland

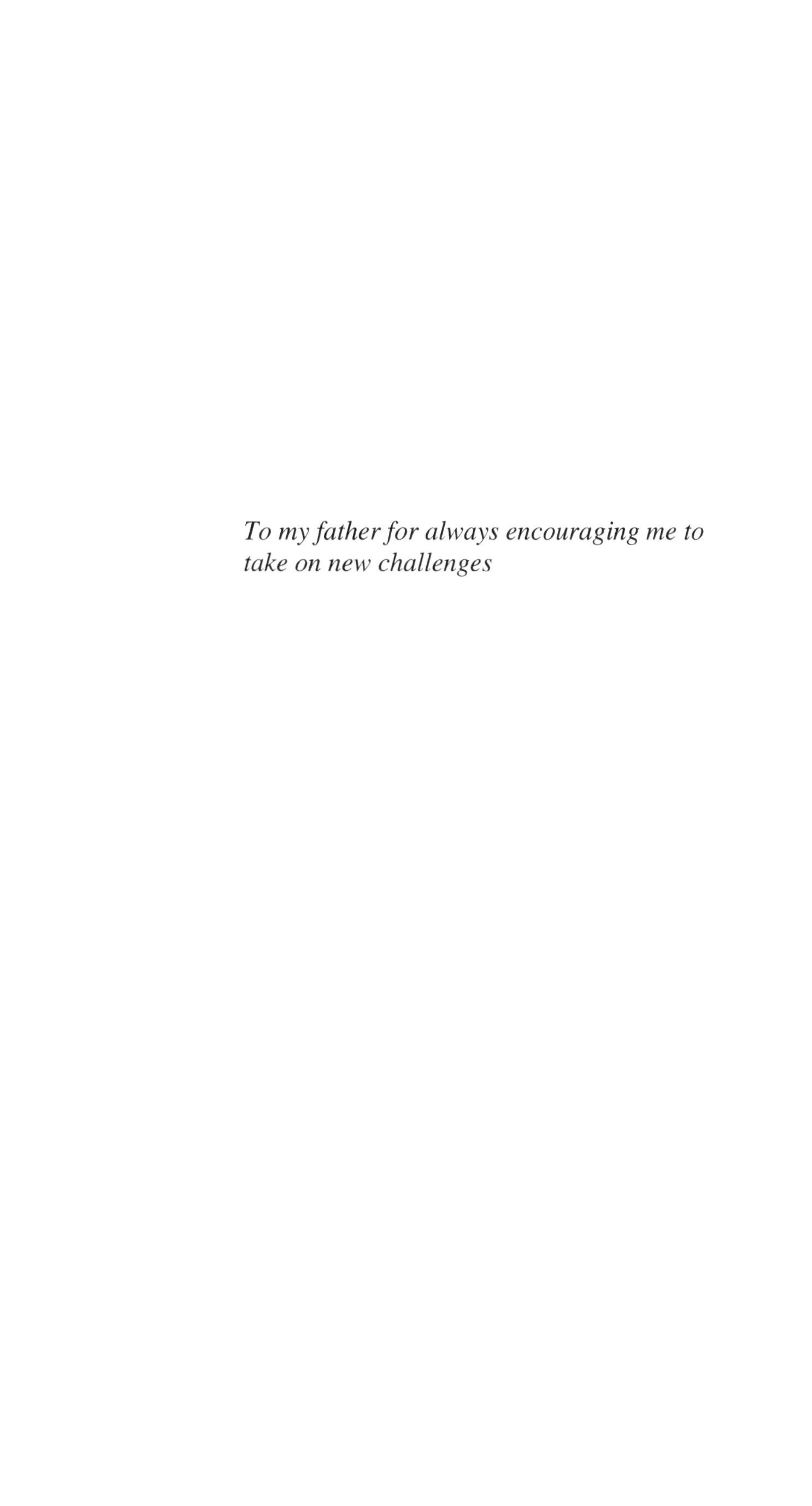

To my father for always encouraging me to take on new challenges

Preface

People with mental illness are faced with many challenges, not the least of which is tolerating the adverse effects of prescribed medications. Like any other category of pharmaceuticals, psychotropic medications have clear benefits but also carry a risk of unwanted side effects. These side effects may be merely a nuisance (e.g., sialorrhea) or they may contribute to the known early mortality in people with mental illness (e.g., obesity). While there are many reasons for the poor health of our patients, the burden of medication-related effects certainly has a role.

Regardless of the intensity and duration of a side effect, any unwanted effect is a burden. As physicians, we strive to minimize these effects for our patients. Our armamentarium of medications for psychiatric illnesses has steadily increased over the last half century, and they are now often a part of treatment along with other critical therapeutic interventions. Psychiatric practitioners are prescribing more medications than ever before.

Psychiatric prescribers have varying degrees of comfort in treating "medical" conditions. There is a movement within psychiatric education to enhance knowledge and skills in primary care for psychiatric prescribers. The degree to which this should occur is a matter of debate. Regardless of intent, actual practice will vary considerably depending on local capabilities and resources. At the very least, prescribers should be able to address the physical health consequences of the medications they prescribe. At one extreme, this may be prescribing medications to treat elevated blood sugar caused by a psychotropic medication. Or it may simply be seeking appropriate consultation for co-management of elevated prolactin from a psychotropic medication. Whether the clinician provides direct treatment or makes a referral, informed decision-making is important.

As a dually trained internist and psychiatrist at our community mental health center, I am often asked questions on managing physical health effects of psychotropic medications. This book is a compilation of symptoms or conditions that I have often encountered either directly or through other providers. Many common conditions unrelated to medications also arise in practice such as new complaints of a respiratory illness or urinary tract infection. While the ability to skillfully triage these conditions is essential to a physician, a discussion of these topics is beyond the scope of this book.

While the focus of the book is medications, it is not a textbook of psychopharmacology. It is not a review of psychotropic medication efficacy in psychiatric illnesses or even a compilation of adverse effects. Rather, the topics center on particular side effects with the emphasis on management approaches. I have attempted to provide a framework for a prescribing clinician to approach medical conditions that result from psychotropic treatment. The intent is to help psychiatric prescribers think as a general practitioner might when approaching these medical conditions. The book is framed for outpatient, long-term care. The recommendations for management assume a lower level of resources such as would be normally expected in an outpatient treatment setting.

While this book is targeted at psychiatric prescribers, primary care practitioners, who frequently prescribe psychotropic medications, may also find it useful. Each chapter lists medications with high and low likelihood of causing a particular side effect. In addition to serving as a reference for clinicians, the book can serve as a curricular aid for psychopharmacology training for psychiatry residents.

I have chosen topics that are clinically relevant and not taught in depth in standard psychopharmacology training. While I do not believe there is a clear distinction between "medical" and "psychiatric" symptoms, I have omitted discussion of "psychiatric" effects that prescribers normally have expertise in (e.g., anxiety, insomnia). I have not included symptoms that occur transiently during treatment (e.g., nausea, headache). While I have not reviewed all rare adverse effects, I have included some that are rare complications of medications but commonly encountered in practice due to other causes (e.g., peripheral edema).

Each chapter follows a similar format except the first chapter on medically ill patients and smaller chapters in the last section. Each of the other chapters contains sections on pathophysiology, etiology, psychotropic medications causing that symptom or condition, clinical features, diagnostic testing, and treatment strategies. Recommendations for treatment are based on evidence when available, expert opinion, and personal clinical experience. Recommendations include thresholds for consultation. Each chapter has highlighted boxes to summarize key learning points and flowcharts to aid decision-making. Key references are listed after each chapter for those interested in further details. I hope these features will make the content easily readable and accessible for busy clinicians.

Psychiatrists are physicians first and specialists second. And nowhere is that more relevant than in psychotropic prescribing. The goal of this book is to help psychiatric practitioners understand the pathophysiology of side effects, formulate a thoughtful differential diagnosis, and develop a management plan that may include seeking an informed consultation. I hope this book will bridge the seemingly disparate realms of psychopharmacologic treatment and general medical care.

New Haven, CT   Aniyizhai Annamalai

Acknowledgments

I am grateful to Cenk Tek, M.D., a friend and colleague who has been instrumental in shaping this book. When I first undertook this project, my goal was to put together a manuscript that would bridge the interface of psychiatry and general medicine by introducing a medical approach to psychotropic prescribing. But the challenge was in presenting the material in a format that was both informative and concise. It was after one particularly illuminating conversation with him that the book started to take on its present format and structure. I still remember that afternoon when we perused several books to identify characteristics that were particularly useful and those that were less than helpful. He reviewed many initial chapters during the early developmental stages of the book. He also provided his expert opinion on many psychopharmacology questions that do not have a clear evidence-based answer. I am thankful for all his contributions.

I want to thank Susan Parke, M.D., and John Cahill, M.D., who reviewed two of the early chapters and provided critical and detailed feedback as clinicians and educators. I want to acknowledge the Yale psychiatry residents whose insightful questions during my lectures on physical health helped me identify gaps in content.

I want to thank my publishers at Springer Science + Business Media who have patiently waited through many iterations of this manuscript.

Finally, I want to thank my family who has been my primary support in all my personal and professional endeavors. My parents are my champions. My sister was my emotional rock during stressful times of writing. My husband was my constant cheerleader and patiently bore my absence during several weekends of busy writing to complete the book.

Contents

Section VI   Genitourinary System

Section VII   Oral and Gastrointestinal System

Section I
Psychotropic Prescribing in Medically Ill Patients

Chapter 1
Psychotropic Prescribing in Medically Ill Patients

This chapter is an overview of general principles of prescribing psychotropic medications in people with preexisting medical conditions. Effects of failure in major organ systems that affect drug absorption, metabolism, and excretion are reviewed.

General Principles

Whenever a new psychotropic medication is prescribed or a patient's physical health condition changes while on chronic psychotropic treatment, the following factors should be considered.

- Can the underlying medical illness cause or exacerbate the presenting psychiatric symptomatology (e.g., hypothyroidism causing fatigue and depression)?
- Do medications used to treat the underlying medical illness have potential for aggravating the psychiatric illness (e.g., corticosteroids and depression, mania or psychosis)?
- Can the underlying medical condition affect the availability, metabolism, or elimination of the psychotropic medication (e.g., reduction of drug absorption after bariatric surgery, changes in protein binding in pregnancy, reduction of drug elimination in end-stage liver disease)?
- Does any underlying genetic variability affect drug metabolism (e.g., more whites than other races are poor metabolizers of CYP2D6 an enzyme that metabolizes many psychotropic medications; more people of Southeast Asian descent have a particular variation of the major histocompatibility complex gene

© Springer International Publishing AG 2017
A. Annamalai, *Medical Management of Psychotropic Side Effects*,
DOI 10.1007/978-3-319-51026-2_1

(HLA-B), namely, HLA-B* 1502, that increases risk for Steven–Johnsons syndrome or toxic epidermal necrolysis when treated with carbamazepine)?
- Does the psychotropic medication cause harm to the underlying or newly developed medical condition (e.g., atypical antipsychotics and diabetes; drugs with teratogenic potential and pregnancy)?
- Do the medications used to treat the medical illness interact with the psychotropic medication causing (a) change in serum level of an agent with a narrow therapeutic index (e.g., lithium toxicity with lithium and diuretics), (b) a serious adverse reaction during combination therapy (e.g., serotonin syndrome with a serotonergic antidepressant and triptans), and (c) loss of efficacy of medication (e.g., decreased efficacy of both phenytoin and carbamazepine when used in combination).

The appendix lists common psychiatric adverse effects of nonpsychotropic medications as well as common drug–drug interactions between psychotropic and nonpsychotropic medications.

Liver Disease

Liver disease affects drug pharmacokinetics in the following ways.

- Decreased synthesis of plasma proteins leading to higher free drug plasma levels
- Decreased liver enzyme synthesis leading to impaired drug metabolism
- Decreased blood flow to liver leading to reduced drug elimination
- Peripheral edema leading to increased volume of distribution
- Vascular congestion and portal hypertension leading to decreased absorption of orally administered drugs

Among all these pathways, decreased liver enzyme synthesis is what causes significant change in psychotropic drug pharmacokinetics. A majority of psychotropic medications are metabolized and excreted through the liver. Hence, with a decrease in liver enzyme synthesis, drug metabolism is reduced requiring a reduction in dose of many psychotropic medications. The table lists the few medications not metabolized in the liver.

Psychotropic drugs not metabolized by the liver

Lithium
Gabapentin
Pregabalin
Topiramate

Liver metabolizes drugs through two phases. Phase I metabolism produces active metabolites from parent drugs by oxidation, reduction, or hydrolysis. Cytochrome P450 is the major isoenzyme family metabolizing the majority of psychotropic medications and the two main isoenzymes are CYP3A4 and CYP2D6.

Phase II metabolism prepares drug products for elimination by glucuronidation, acetylation, or sulfation. The major family of enzymes involved in psychotropic drug metabolism is the uridine glucuronyltransferases (mainly 2B7). Phase II metabolism is generally preserved in liver cirrhosis. Some medications that undergo almost exclusively phase II metabolism are lorazepam, oxazepam, and temazepam [1]. These benzodiazepines are preferentially used in patients with liver disease.

There are many substances, including prescribed medications, that affect P450 activity and thus alter levels of other drugs. Some common P450 inhibitors and inducers, including psychotropic medications, are listed in the table.

Substances affecting P450 activity

P450 inhibitors (increase medication levels)
Ketoconazole (2C9)
Amiodarone (1A2, 2C9, 2D6)
Isoniazid (2C19)
Diltiazem (3A4)
Grape fruit juice (1A2, 3A4)
Omeprazole (2C19)
Many protease inhibitors (3A4)
Quinidine (2D6)
Ciprofloxacin (1A2)
Fluoxetine (2C9)
Fluvoxamine (1A2)
Paroxetine (2D6)
Ritonavir (2C9, 2C19, 2D6, 3A4)
P450 inducers (decrease medication levels)
Rifampin (2C9, 2C19)
Phenytoin (2C9, 2C19)
Carbamazepine (1A2, 2C9, 2C19)
St. Johns wort (3A4)
Cigarette smoking (polycyclic aromatic hydrocarbons) (1A1, 1A2)

Medications with long half-lives, active metabolites, and extended release formulations may have less predictable pharmacokinetics and are less preferable in liver disease.

In general, it is prudent to start any medication at a lower dose and titrate slowly in the presence of liver disease. Medications to be used with particular caution are listed in the table.

Psychotropic medication categories to be used with caution in liver disease

Category	Mechanism	Example
Drugs with potential for hepatotoxicity	Carry an increased risk with preexisting liver disease	Carbamazepine, valproate, duloxetine
Drugs with sedative and anticholinergic properties	May precipitate hepatic encephalopathy due to intestinal stasis and central effects	Low-potency antipsychotics, benzodiazepines
Drugs at risk for causing cytopenias	May worsen low blood counts seen in liver disease	Carbamazepine, antipsychotics
Long-acting medications	Generally have less predictable pharmacokinetics	Extended release formulations

Renal Disease

Renal disease affects drug pharmacokinetics in the following ways.

- Decreased clearance of active drug or metabolites
- Increased volume of distribution
- Decreased albumin level and reduced availability of plasma-binding proteins
- Indirectly by effect on hepatic metabolism

Very few psychotropic medications need significant dosage adjustment in renal failure but, in general, it is prudent to reduce medication doses. Medications of particular concern are listed in the table.

Psychotropic medication categories to be used with caution in renal disease

Category	Mechanism	Example
Medications excreted by kidney	Potential for toxic blood levels	Lithium, gabapentin, pregabalin, topiramate
Medications whose active metabolites are partially excreted by kidney	May need dose reduction due to decreased clearance	Bupropion, venlafaxine, desvenlafaxine, mirtazapine, risperidone, paliperidone, paroxetine
Medications that are protein bound	May need dose reduction due to reduced plasma-binding proteins	Valproate
Medications with risk of arrhythmia	May have higher risk of adverse effect due to coexisting electrolyte imbalance	Any medication that increases risk for QTc prolongation

Most psychotropic medications are lipophilic and have a large volume of distribution and are not easily excreted on dialysis. Medications that are hydrophilic (e.g., lithium, gabapentin) are easily dialyzed out and can be used in patients on hemodialysis. Other psychotropic medications may be dialyzable with high permeability hemodialysis [2]. Dialyzability of medications depends on many factors and decisions on using them in patients on dialysis have to be made with the treating nephrologist.

Neurologic Disease

Stroke

Some medications may exacerbate symptoms seen in patients with prior strokes. The following are key points to remember when prescribing for patients with history of stroke.

- Use agents likely to cause orthostatic hypotension with caution
- Use selective serotonin reuptake inhibitors (SSRIs) with caution if also on anticoagulants though risk of cerebral bleeding is small
- Use all antipsychotics with caution in patients with dementia as they carry a warning for risk of stroke

Seizures

Many psychotropic medications lower seizure threshold but absolute risk at therapeutic doses is small. Medications with a slightly higher risk are clozapine, chlorpromazine, tricyclic antidepressants, and bupropion. These medications are not contraindicated in those with seizure disorder but are preferably avoided as first-line agents. If they are used, medication-related risk factors including rapid titration, high doses, and rapid withdrawal should be minimized.

There is a more detailed discussion of seizures and psychotropic medications in Chapter 41.

Cardiovascular Disease

Some medications may exacerbate symptoms seen in patients with cardiovascular disease. Examples of some common adverse effects are listed in the table.

Additive risk of psychotropic medication effects and cardiac conditions

Category	Conditions increasing risk	Examples
Medications that cause conduction abnormalities (prolonged QTc or atrioventricular conduction)	Bradycardia, congestive heart failure, myocardial infarction, mitral valve prolapse	Many antipsychotics, tricyclic antidepressants (TCAs), lithium
Medications that cause orthostatic hypotension	Left ventricular failure from myocardial infarction or other causes	TCAs, low-potency antipsychotics
Medications that increase heart rate, blood pressure	Congestive heart failure, diastolic dysfunction from chronic hypertension	Clozapine, some antidepressants, some stimulants

Also, congestive heart failure can cause peripheral edema and affect volume of distribution of medications. It also may result in reduced cardiac output and decreased hepatic blood flow. Heart failure may also cause renal dysfunction and indirectly affect drug excretion.

Respiratory Disease

Dosage adjustments for psychotropic medications are generally not necessary in respiratory illness. Cystic fibrosis may cause some changes in drug absorption and hepatic metabolism. Hydrocarbons in tobacco smoke reduce levels of medications that are metabolized by the CYP1A2 pathway (e.g., clozapine, olanzapine).

Some medications should be used in caution in patients with respiratory disease. Some key points are listed as follows.

- Benzodiazepines suppress respiratory drive

  - They are generally not preferred in obstructive pulmonary disease but can be used if significant anxiety interferes with respiration
  - If benzodiazepines are used, intermediate-acting agents are better
  - Benzodiazepines should be avoided, if possible, in obstructive sleep apnea

- Beta blockers for anxiety are not contraindicated but should be used in caution in patients with asthma (e.g., propranolol)

Gastrointestinal Disease

Generally, medication pharmacokinetics is not affected by gastrointestinal disease except in some select conditions.

- Bariatric surgery may alter medication kinetics by affecting drug absorption and volume of distribution via loss of adipose tissue

  - If surgery includes malabsorptive procedures like the Roux-en-Y bypass, it results in reduced absorption of most medications
  - Bupropion and lithium are exceptions with increased levels seen after bypass surgery [3]
  - Patients should be monitored for continued efficacy of medications after gastric bypass
  - In general, liquid formulations, orally disintegrating medicines, and immediate release formulations are more likely to produce steady plasma levels after bypass surgery

- Celiac disease may reduce absorption of medications

There is a small risk of gastric bleeding with selective serotonergic reuptake inhibitors (SSRIs) in people with gastric erosions (see Chapter 27 for a more detailed discussion). If possible, medications with anticholinergic effect should be avoided in people with gastroparesis. If patient has a motility disorder that causes diarrhea, SSRIs may exacerbate this symptom.

Pregnancy

Factors affecting medication pharmacokinetics in pregnancy are changes in drug–protein binding, increased volume of distribution, and increased renal filtration. The last two factors may necessitate an increased dose of medications in late pregnancy.

The decision of whether to continue psychotropic medication during pregnancy is individualized. A detailed discussion of teratogenicity of individual drugs is beyond the scope of this book. The appendix lists commonly known adverse effects of psychotropic medications in pregnancy.

Medication Use in Lactation

Medications are variably excreted in breast milk and recommendations are individualized for each agent. Generally agents with sedating properties carry a risk of neonatal sedation. Medications with shorter half-lives are preferred to minimize this effect. There is a theoretical risk of common or serious adverse effects of some medications passing on to the neonate (e.g., lithium and hypothyroidism, clozapine and agranulocytosis).

Appendix

Selected psychiatric adverse effects of nonpsychotropic medications [4]

Medication class	Adverse effect
Steroids	Dose-dependent risk of depression, mania and rarely, psychosis
Hormonal contraceptives	Risk of depression, mood instability, especially with higher progestin content
Opiates	Associated with acute delirium and psychosis
Varenicline	Case reports of depression and suicidal ideation but not replicated in large cohorts
Beta blockers	Associated with depression but low risk; not replicated in large cohorts
Anticonvulsants	Delirium and psychosis, possibly depression
Interferon	High risk of depression (less commonly used now with advent of directly acting antiviral agents for hepatitis C)
Antiretroviral medications (e.g., efavirenz, zidovudine)	Depression, suicidal ideation, personality changes

Selected psychotropic and nonpsychotropic drug interactions

Psychotropic	Interaction with nonpsychotropic
Lithium	Thiazide diuretics, nonsteroidal anti-inflammatory drugs (NSAIDs) increase lithium concentration by tubal reabsorption
Benzodiazepines	Opiate concurrent use carries risk of severe respiratory suppression
Selective serotonin reuptake inhibitors (SSRIs)	Serotonergic agents (e.g., triptans, tramadol, opiates) use increases risk for serotonin syndrome
Antipsychotics that increase risk of QTc prolongation	Antibiotics (e.g., quinolones, macrolide agents) carry additive risk
Low-potency antipsychotics, tricyclic antidepressants (TCAs)	Antihypertensives, especially multiple agents, increase risk for orthostasis
Carbamazepine	Phenytoin decreases medication level and some medications (e.g., macrolide antibiotics, azole antifungals, isoniazid) increase medication level Oral contraceptive levels and efficacy may be lowered when used with carbamazepine

Psychotropic medications and pregnancy [5, 6]

Medication class	Effects in pregnancy
Antidepressants	Low risk of teratogenicity with all classes Selective serotonergic reuptake inhibitors (SSRIs) associated with increased risk of premature birth, neonatal pulmonary hypertension though extent of risk is small Paroxetine possibly carries higher risk
Antipsychotics	Low risk of teratogenicity Some risk of gestational diabetes and related complications Possible neonatal sedation and transient extrapyramidal symptoms
Mood stabilizers	Risk of Ebstein's anomaly with lithium is low; possible risk of neonatal hypothyroidism Carbamazepine and valproate associated with significant risk of neural tube defects and are relatively contraindicated Lamotrigine is likely the safest agent in this category
Benzodiazepines	Low risk of teratogenicity Possible sedation and neonatal withdrawal syndrome
Stimulants	Low risk of teratogenicity Possible premature birth, low birth weight, neonatal withdrawal syndrome

References

1. Nair B. Psychopharmacology in medically ill patients. In: Leigh H, Streltzer J, editors. Handbook of consultation-liaison psychiatry. 2nd ed. New York: Springer International Publishing; 2015.
2. Owen JA, Levenson JL. Renal and urological disorders. In: Ferrando SJ, Levenson JL, Owen JA, editors. Clinical manual of psychopharmacology in the medically ill. 1st ed. Wahington, DC: American Psychiatric Publishing; 2010.
3. Crone CC, Marcangelo M, Lackamp J, DiMartini AF, Owen JA. Gastrointestinal disorders. In: Ferrando SJ, Levenson JL, Owen JA, editors. Clinical manual of psychopharmacology of the medically ill. 1st ed. Washington, DC: American Psychiatric Publishing; 2010.
4. Turjanski NLG. Psychiatric side-effects of medications: recent developments. Adv Psych Treat. 2005;11(1):58–70.
5. Kohen D. Psychotropic medication in pregnancy. Adv Psych Treat. 2003;10(1):59–66.
6. Altemus A, Occhiogrosso M. Obstetrics and gynecology. In: Ferrando SJ, Levenson JL, Owen JA, editors. Clinical manual of psychopharmacology in the medically ill. Washington, DC: American Psychiatric Publishing; 2010.

Section II
Metabolic Syndrome

Chapter 2
Obesity

Metabolic syndrome refers to a group of conditions that increase risk for cardiovascular disease. It includes obesity, diabetes, hypertension, and abnormal lipids.

Obesity, defined by a body mass index (BMI) >30 kg/m^2, is associated with increased morbidity and mortality. The prevalence of obesity is >30% of the U.S. general population and >50% in people with serious mental illness [1]. A BMI >25 kg/m^2 is considered overweight and is also a risk factor for many diseases.

Pathology

An increase in body fat results from a higher energy intake than expenditure. However, many factors mediate the food intake and energy balance and weight gain is not a simple calculation of intake minus expenditure. Several gut peptides, including leptin and ghrelin, are involved in regulation of hunger and satiety. Also, with age, the decline in reproductive hormones predisposes to weight gain.

Etiology

A genetic predisposition coupled with a lifestyle that promotes unhealthy diets and lack of physical activity is the most common cause of obesity. Much less commonly, secondary causes such as hypothyroidism, Cushing's syndrome, and polycystic ovarian syndrome cause weight gain.

© Springer International Publishing AG 2017

A. Annamalai, *Medical Management of Psychotropic Side Effects*,

DOI 10.1007/978-3-319-51026-2_2

In patients with serious mental illness, psychotropic medications contribute significantly to weight gain. Socioeconomic factors and unhealthy lifestyle habits are additional factors.

Psychotropic Medications and Obesity

Many psychotropic agents cause weight gain as a side effect. Many mechanisms are thought to contribute to increased appetite, including central histamine (H1) blockade, serotonin (5HT2c) blockade, and dopamine (D2) blockade.

Most antipsychotics induce some degree of weight gain. Weight gain is more pronounced in medication-naïve patients. For instance, haloperidol, thought to be relatively weight neutral in patients with chronic illness, causes weight gain when used in medication-naïve patients [2]. Clozapine and olanzapine carry highest risk while ziprasidone carries the least risk of weight gain [2, 3]. Low-potency typical antipsychotics like chlorpromazine carry a significant risk of weight gain. Weight increases exponentially in the first months of antipsychotic treatment. In clinical experience, the maximal gain appears to be in the first 1–2 years though it can continue in later years also. There is no consistent evidence of a relationship between antipsychotic dose and risk of weight gain.

Antidepressants also can cause weight gain. Notable examples are mirtazapine and tricyclic antidepressants (TCAs) [4]. Evidence on extent of weight gain with selective serotonin reuptake inhibitors (SSRIs) and serotonin norepinephrine reuptake inhibitors (SNRIs) is variable across studies [4, 5]. Mood stabilizers such as lithium and valproate also cause weight gain though to a lesser extent than antipsychotics. Antihistamines when used consistently also can induce weight gain.

The following table categorizes psychotropic medications into approximate risk categories.

Psychotropic medications and propensity to weight gain

	Most likely	Intermediate	Least likely
Antipsychotics	Clozapine, olanzapine, chlorpromazine	Risperidone, paliperidone, quetiapine, haloperidol[a]	Ziprasidone, lurasidone, aripiprazole, perphenazine, asenapine, fluphenazine
Mood stabilizers	Valproate, lithium	Carbamazepine, oxcarbazepine	Lamotrigine
Antidepressants	TCAs, monoamine oxidase inhibitors, (MAOIs), mirtazapine	Paroxetine	Sertraline, citalopram, escitalopram, venlafaxine, duloxetine Note: Both bupropion and fluoxetine cause some weight loss, though effect is primarily in acute treatment phase for fluoxetine

[a]Haloperidol shows weight gain when used as early intervention but not in patients on maintenance treatment

> ***Almost all antipsychotics, including typical agents, are associated with some weight gain.***
>
> ***There is no clear relationship between dose of antipsychotic and effect on weight.***

Clinical Features

Besides the psychological effects and stigma of increased weight, the clinical manifestations of obesity result from its medical complications. Major complications include diabetes mellitus, dyslipidemia, coronary artery disease, and obstructive sleep apnea. Obesity also is a risk factor for liver disease, gall stone formation, osteoarthritis, fractures, skin infections, and some malignancies.

> ***The main clinical consequences of obesity are those related to its complications.***

Diagnosis

BMI is the first measure to determine unhealthy weight. It is calculated as body weight (kg)/height (meters) squared. Standard cutoff values may not be reliable in elderly, those with increased muscle mass, and in certain races. See table for weight and BMI categories.

Weight classification by BMI (in kg/m²)

Underweight	<18.5
Normal weight	18.5–24.9
Overweight	25–29.9
Obesity class I	30–34.9
Obesity class II	35–39.9
Obesity class III	≥40

Waist circumference is an additional tool to estimate risk from increased fat mass. It is most useful in a midrange of BMI 25–35 kg/m² as it does not add much predictive value at higher BMIs. It can also be useful in Asian populations where abdominal fat is a better indicator of metabolic risk than BMI. Waist circumference is measured with a tape placed horizontally around the abdominal wall at the level of the iliac crest. Abdominal adiposity independently increases risk of weight-related complications. The cutoff range for men and women is shown in the table.

Abnormal waist circumference

Men	>40 in. or 102 cm
Women	>35 in. or 88 cm

Beyond establishing at-risk weight, the workup for obesity is evaluating comorbid conditions, especially metabolic risk factors such as diabetes, hypertension, and dyslipidemia. Additional testing may be done if symptoms and signs indicate secondary etiologies like hypothyroidism.

> *Waist circumference is useful as an additional prognostic tool especially when BMI is in the overweight range (25–30 kg/m2)*

Management

The first and most important step in managing obesity due to psychotropic medications is selecting weight neutral medications or those that even cause some weight loss. Often, medications that carry risk for weight gain may need to be used but they should not be used as first-line agents. Antipsychotics especially should not be used as initial augmenting agents for treatment of mood disorders.

When weight gain has already occurred, medication should be switched unless clinically infeasible. Any weight gain, especially over the normal range, increases risk of complications and medication switch should be considered. It is strongly recommended if weight continues to rise, especially if more than 5% gain has occurred. There is evidence that weight loss occurs on switching from other antipsychotics to ziprasidone or aripiprazole [6]. If a switch is not possible or if weight does not decrease even after the switch, aggressive treatment for the weight gain should be initiated. Decreasing antipsychotic dose can be tried but success in weight reduction is equivocal.

Weight measurement and discussion of lifestyle changes should occur at every visit. Weight measurement should occur at least every 6 weeks in the first 6 months of treatment. If weight is stable, it can then be measured every 3–6 months. Education on lifestyle modification includes identifying high calorie diets in food, incorporating more physical activity into the daily routine, and reducing triggers such as emotional eating. Setting very specific targets (e.g., reducing one sugary drink per week) is more likely to be effective than general advice. Whenever available, a structured lifestyle intervention program should be implemented. Even a 5% weight reduction carries substantial gains in cardiovascular risk reduction.

A medication can be considered along with lifestyle interventions, especially when significant weight gain has occurred with antipsychotics. Metformin has shown good evidence in weight gain induced by antipsychotics. It may be especially appropriate in those who develop prediabetes. Topiramate has shown some efficacy in patients on antipsychotics but has cognitive side effects. The phentermine/topiramate combination is generally avoided due to risk of psychosis exacerbation with phentermine. Naltrexone/bupropion combination holds promise and is being studied for weight loss in people on antipsychotics. Other FDA-approved medications (orlistat, lorcaserin) have not been well studied in this population. Bariatric surgery should be offered to patients with class III obesity and class II obesity with medical complications. Throughout treatment, patients should be monitored for obesity-related conditions such as diabetes, hypertension, hyperlipidemia.

See Appendix for list of weight loss medications as well as indications for bariatric surgery.

Evidence for strategies to slow or stop psychotropic-induced weight gain exists mostly for antipsychotics. The same strategies of switching medications and instituting structured lifestyle interventions should be attempted for all medications that cause weight gain.

Initiating or switching to more weight neutral medications is key to managing medication-induced weight gain.

Structured lifestyle interventions should be implemented for all patients with weight gain; weight loss medications can be considered.

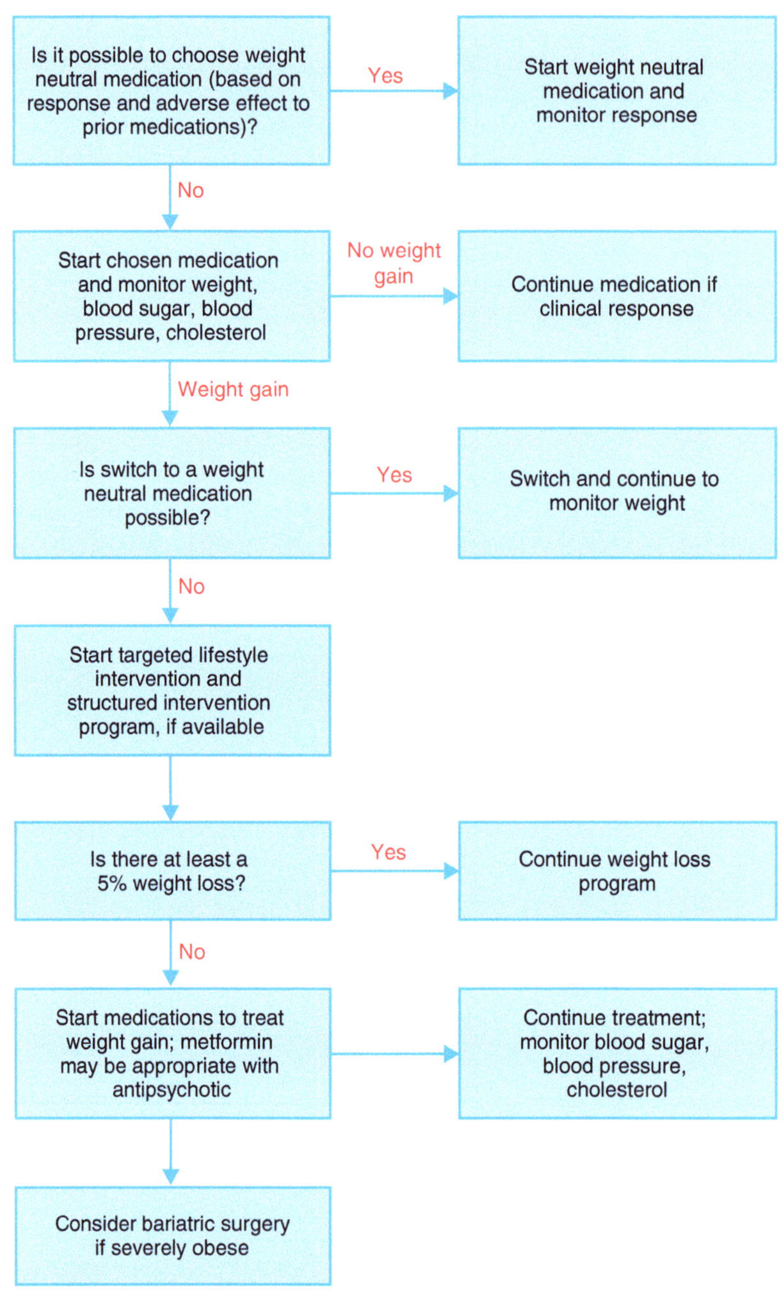
Is it possible to choose weight neutral medication (based on response and adverse effect to prior medications)?
Yes
Start weight neutral medication and monitor response
No
Start chosen medication and monitor weight, blood sugar, blood pressure, cholesterol
No weight gain
Continue medication if clinical response
Weight gain
Is switch to a weight neutral medication possible?
Yes
Switch and continue to monitor weight
No
Start targeted lifestyle intervention and structured intervention program, if available
Is there at least a 5% weight loss?
Yes
Continue weight loss program
No
Start medications to treat weight gain; metformin may be appropriate with antipsychotic
Continue treatment; monitor blood sugar, blood pressure, cholesterol
Consider bariatric surgery if severely obese

Appendix

Weight loss medications approved by FDA[a]

Medication	Mechanism	Side effects
Phentermine/topiramate	Phentermine is a sympathomimetic amine and reduces appetite; topiramate acts on multiple receptors to reduce food craving	Poor memory and concentration, xerostomia, tachycardia; potential to worsen psychosis
Orlistat	Inhibits pancreatic lipase and intestinal fat absorption	Oily stools, flatus, fecal urgency,
Lorcaserin	5H2Tc agonist; stimulates release of melanocortin that reduces appetite	Headache, nausea, dizziness
Naltrexone/bupropion[b]	Bupropion stimulates hypothalamic neurons that reduce appetite; naltrexone blocks beta-endorphin and increases anorexigenic effect	Nausea, constipation, insomnia
Liraglutide	Glucagon-like peptide (GLP-1) agonist that reduces appetite by central and peripheral pathways	Rarely, pancreatitis, medullary thyroid carcinoma; small risk of suicidal ideation

[a]These medications have limited or no evidence for weight loss in people with mental illness
[b]Naltrexone has emerging but, as yet limited evidence for people with mental illness; bupropion is known to cause modest weight loss in depression studies

Indications for bariatric surgery[a] based on National Institute of Health (NIH) guidelines[b]

Class III obesity (BMI >40 kg/m^2) even without comorbidities
Class II obesity (BMI 35–39.9 kg/m^2) and at least one medical complication (e.g., diabetes mellitus, obstructive sleep apnea)

[a]There is evidence for successful outcomes in people with mental illness; prior to referral, psychiatric illness should be well controlled and there should not be active substance abuse
[b]In addition to listed indications, it can be considered for class I obesity (BMI 30–34.9 kg/m^2) with uncontrolled type 2 diabetes mellitus, especially in Asian populations

References

1. Correll CU, Druss BG, Lombardo I, O'Gorman C, Harnett JP, Sanders KN, et al. Findings of a U.S. national cardiometabolic screening program among 10,084 psychiatric outpatients. Psychiatr Serv. 2010;61(9):892–8.
2. Tek C, Kucukgoncu S, Guloksuz S, Woods SW, Srihari VH, Annamalai A. Antipsychotic-induced weight gain in first-episode psychosis patients: a meta-analysis of differential effects of antipsychotic medications. Early Interv Psychiatry. 2016;10(3):193–202.
3. Leucht S, Cipriani A, Spineli L, Mavridis D, Orey D, Richter F, et al. Comparative efficacy and tolerability of 15 antipsychotic drugs in schizophrenia: a multiple-treatments meta-analysis. Lancet. 2013;382(9896):951–62.
4. Serretti A, Mandelli L. Antidepressants and body weight: a comprehensive review and meta-analysis. J Clin Psychiatry. 2010;71(10):1259–72.
5. Uguz F, Sahingoz M, Gungor B, Aksoy F, Askin R. Weight gain and associated factors in patients using newer antidepressant drugs. Gen Hosp Psychiatry. 2015;37(1):46–8.
6. Wieden PJ, Newcomer JW. Evidence of switching antipsychotic therapy to improve metabolic disturbances. J Clin Psychiatry. 2007;68(5):e13.

Chapter 3
Diabetes Mellitus and Acute Hyperglycemia

Diabetes mellitus (DM) prevalence is reported as high as 10% in the general population and is even higher in those with mental illness. An elevated blood sugar is seen in almost 20% patients with serious mental illness [1]. The cutoffs for accepted and commonly used measures to diagnose DM are shown in the section on diagnosis later.

Acute hyperglycemia is seen with two conditions associated with DM—diabetic ketoacidosis and hyperosmolar coma.

Pathology

The pathophysiology of DM is complicated. There are varying degrees of insulin deficiency and peripheral resistance to the action of insulin. Genetic susceptibility and environmental factors together lead to DM development. Hyperglycemia itself worsens insulin resistance leading to slow progression of DM.

Etiology

Weight gain and decreased physical activity are two major risk factors that promote DM development. Among nonpsychotropic medications that cause hyperglycemia, corticosteroids are a notable example. DM is often associated with other medical conditions that increase risk for cardiovascular disease. The constellation of obesity, diabetes, hypertension, and elevated lipids is termed metabolic syndrome.

© Springer International Publishing AG 2017

A. Annamalai, *Medical Management of Psychotropic Side Effects*,
DOI 10.1007/978-3-319-51026-2_3

Psychotropic Medications and Hyperglycemia

Antipsychotics, especially those with increased propensity to cause metabolic syndrome, increase risk for hyperglycemia. While much of the effect is related to development of obesity, it is thought that antipsychotics may independently impair glucose regulation. One proposed mechanism is via blocking the muscarinic pancreatic receptor. The risk is increased both for developing chronic DM and an acute hyperglycemic episode. Hyperglycemia can develop as early as within 4 weeks of starting an antipsychotic; the mean duration is about 19 weeks of exposure [2]. This acute hyperglycemic effect may also reflect unmasking of underlying susceptibility to diabetes mellitus.

The same agents that increase risk for obesity increase risk of hyperglycemia and metabolic syndrome. Clozapine and olanzapine carry the highest risk. As a group, typical antipsychotics carry an equivalent risk to atypical antipsychotics when clozapine and olanzapine are excluded from the latter group [3].

Antipsychotics are also associated with acute hyperglycemic episodes. Older age is a risk factor. In addition to clozapine and olanzapine, risperidone and quetiapine are associated with numerous cases of acute hyperglycemia [2, 4, 5]. There are rare case reports of aripiprazole and diabetic ketoacidosis.

Acute hyperglycemia occurs both as a new diagnosis and exacerbation of preexisting DM. A possible mechanism is direct toxicity to pancreatic islet cells. Patients with preexisting diabetes are placed at higher risk of serious hyperglycemia upon initiation of an antipsychotic. But hyperglycemia can occur even without any history of diabetes and has been documented in patients started on clozapine, olanzapine, quetiapine, and risperidone. It is reversible in some cases. Risk factors that could precipitate acute hyperglycemia are poor fluid intake, substance use, systemic illness, and nonadherence to insulin in those with diagnosed DM.

There is increased hyperglycemia observed with antidepressant therapy but no causal link has been established. Any psychotropic agent that induces weight gain also carries some risk of accompanying DM.

Antipsychotics and propensity to diabetes

	Most likely	Intermediate	Least likely
Antipsychotics	Clozapine, olanzapine	Quetiapine, risperidone, paliperidone, low-potency typical agents	Ziprasidone, lurasidone, aripiprazole, perphenazine, high-potency typical agents

The antipsychotics most likely to cause diabetes mellitus are the same as those that cause weight gain.

Many antipsychotics are also associated with acute onset of hyperglycemia with or without preexisting diabetes mellitus.

Clinical Features

Patients with DM are usually asymptomatic for months or years before hyperglycemia becomes severe. They may then present with polyuria, polydipsia, blurred vision, and rarely polyphagia.

Acute hyperglycemia may sometimes occur as the initial manifestation of illness and patients then are acutely ill with symptoms resulting from volume depletion, electrolyte imbalance, and altered mental status.

Poorly controlled DM is associated with complications of skin changes, infections, altered peripheral sensation, visual abnormalities, kidney disease, ischemic heart disease, and stroke.

Clinical features of hyperglycemia

Chronic hyperglycemia	Usually asymptomatic May have polydipsia, polyuria, weight changes In advanced disease, symptoms of organ damage manifest
Acute hyperglycemia	May be asymptomatic but can present as nausea/vomiting, abdominal pain, polyuria, headache, fatigue, altered mental status

Slow development of diabetes mellitus usually has no symptoms until the hyperglycemia becomes severe.

Acute hyperglycemia presents usually with nonspecific symptoms of a systemic illness.

Diagnosis

Hyperglycemia is any elevation of blood sugar above the normal range in healthy individuals. Fasting blood sugar (FBS) or glycosylated hemoglobin (HbA1c) is used to diagnose DM. HbA1c is a measure of the percentage of glucose carried by hemoglobin and does not vary with fasting state. When HbA1c and FBS are discrepant, the higher of the two should be used (e.g., if HbA1c is in the diabetes range and FBS is in the prediabetes range, patient is considered to have DM). The random blood sugar is not as reliable a measure as FBS or HbA1c but values > 200 mg/dL are considered high.

The diagnosis of diabetes is made using criteria shown in the table.

Diagnosis of diabetes

	At-risk for diabetes (prediabetes)	Diabetes
Glycosylated hemoglobin (HbA1c) (%)	5.7–6.4	≥6.5
Fasting blood sugar (FBS) (mg/dL)	100–125	≥126
Random blood glucose (RBS) (mg/dL)	—	≥200 with symptoms

The blood sugar goals in patients with DM depend on age and other risk factors. HbA1c is usually the measure used for monitoring adequacy of treatment while FBS is used to titrate dosage adjustments in those on daily insulin.

Diabetes ketoacidosis (DKA), resulting from near-complete lack of insulin, causes excess ketoacids and blood sugar in the 400–800 mg/dL range. Hyperglycemic hyperosmolar state (HHS), resulting from partial insulin deficiency, causes blood glucose > 1000 mg/dL and very few ketoacids. Metabolic acidosis and high anion gap is more pronounced in DKA and serum osmolality is much higher in HHS.

> **Either HbA1c or FBS can be used to diagnose diabetes mellitus; HbA1c is used to monitor diabetes treatment.**

Management

The key to managing hyperglycemia with psychotropic medications is prevention. Antipsychotics should only be used when there are clear indications. When used, agents at low risk for metabolic syndrome should be selected, whenever possible.

Both DM and acute hyperglycemia are discussed as follows.

Diabetes Mellitus (DM)

Antipsychotics with higher risk for metabolic syndrome should be used only after other options have failed. If a high-risk agent such as olanzapine is necessary for symptom control, some experts recommend adding metformin prophylactically though this is not common practice. Lifestyle factors should be continually addressed to prevent DM onset. Structured interventions to manage weight gain will also prevent or slow development of DM.

In patients who develop prediabetes or diabetes on antipsychotic medication, dose reduction can be tried but it is recommended that the offending agent be stopped unless strongly indicated. It should be noted, however, that the glucose dysregulation might not always be reversible upon cessation of the causative agent. For prediabetes, metformin has some evidence for preventing conversion to diabetes and may be useful in also promoting weight loss. Again, lifestyle modifications should be emphasized. Once DM develops, patients should be referred for long-term management while optimizing antipsychotic treatment. Metformin is first-line agent and may be sufficient if HbA1c <9%. Many oral agents are now available for additional blood sugar control if metformin is insufficient (see Appendix). Insulin often becomes necessary with disease progression.

Metformin can be used in people with mild to moderate kidney disease. It should not be used if GFR <30 mL/min. Dose should be halved for GFR <45 mL/min.

Long-term metformin use is linked to B12 deficiency and so B12 levels should be periodically monitored.

> ***Medication switch and structured lifestyle interventions should be the initial interventions if new onset hyperglycemia occurs; metformin is useful to prevent conversion of prediabetes to diabetes.***

Acute Hyperglycemia

Severe hyperglycemia can manifest acutely as DKA or HHS.

The diagnosis of acute hyperglycemia should be considered in any acutely ill patient newly started on antipsychotics, even if they do not have known DM. If a patient presents with new onset polyuria and polydipsia, blood sugar should be measured. With mild hyperglycemia, there may be nonspecific systemic symptoms like fatigue and poor attention. With significant elevations of blood sugar, there may be additional symptoms such as nausea, vomiting, respiratory difficulties, or changes in cognition.

Intervention depends on presence and severity of symptoms, extent of blood sugar elevation, and whether the hyperglycemia is new or exacerbation of preexisting diabetes. Any patients with symptoms indicative of severe hyperglycemia should receive urgent evaluation for DKA and HHS. Asymptomatic patients with blood sugar <400 mg/dl generally will not need urgent evaluation for DKA or HHS. However, in a patient with no history of diabetes, even a blood sugar over 250 mg/dL may warrant evaluation for DKA or HHS especially if accompanied by mild or nonspecific symptoms. In a patient with known poorly controlled diabetes, a random blood sugar even up to 500 mg/dL may only reflect chronic hyperglycemia and need for urgent evaluation depends on presence of any new symptoms.

Typically blood sugar is 400–800 mg/dL in DKA and >1000 mg/dL in HHS. A urine dipstick test for ketonuria may be useful to test for DKA when blood sugar is relatively low and symptoms are equivocal; however, this is difficult to obtain in most psychiatric settings.

Even though DM related to antipsychotics is not associated with complete insulin deficiency, DKA has been reported more commonly than HHS. After an acute episode of DKA has been appropriately managed, the antipsychotic should be discontinued unless there is a strong indication. Even after stopping the agent, more than half the patients need continued treatment for hyperglycemia [6].

> ***Intervention for acute hyperglycemia depends on presence of symptoms and/or preexisting diabetes.***
>
> ***Hyperglycemia may persist even after offending medication is stopped.***

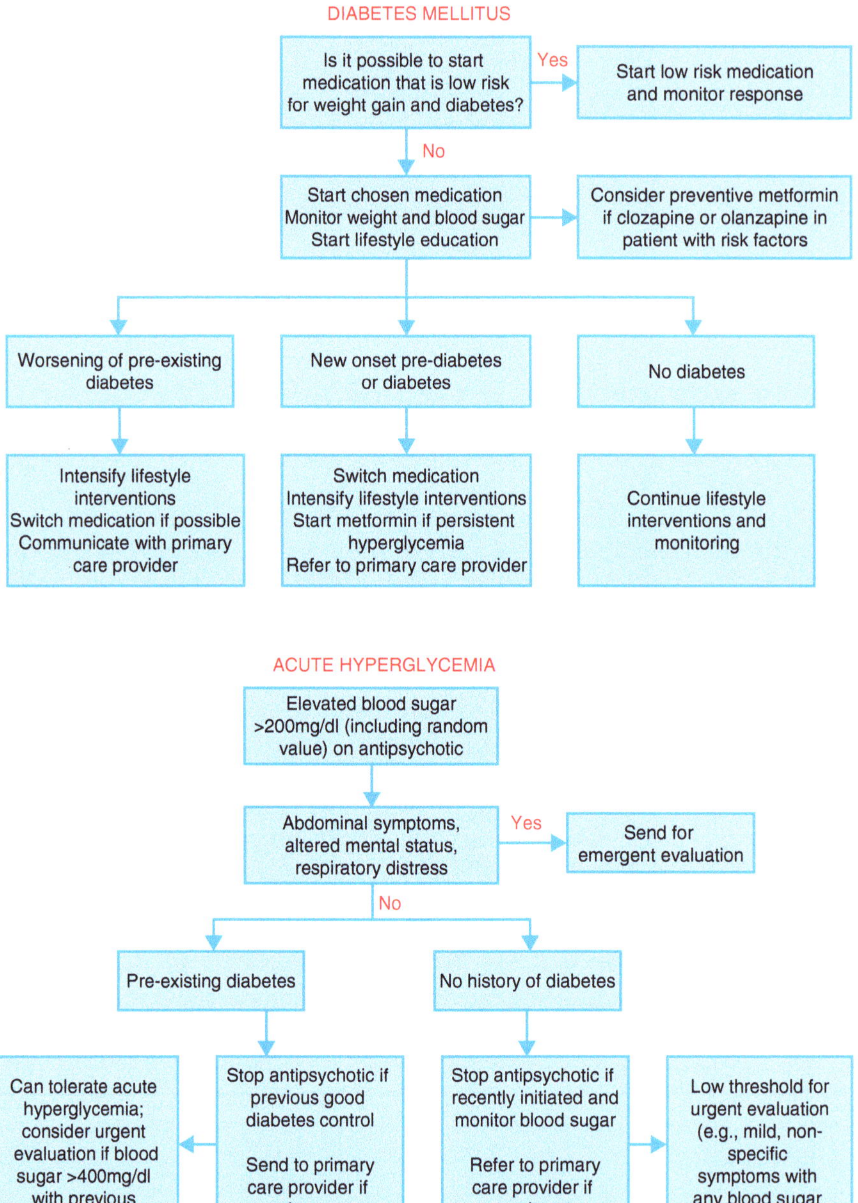
DIABETES MELLITUS

Is it possible to start medication that is low risk for weight gain and diabetes?
Yes
Start low risk medication and monitor response
No
Start chosen medication
Monitor weight and blood sugar
Start lifestyle education
Consider preventive metformin if clozapine or olanzapine in patient with risk factors

Worsening of pre-existing diabetes
New onset pre-diabetes or diabetes
No diabetes

Intensify lifestyle interventions
Switch medication if possible
Communicate with primary care provider

Switch medication
Intensify lifestyle interventions
Start metformin if persistent hyperglycemia
Refer to primary care provider

Continue lifestyle interventions and monitoring

ACUTE HYPERGLYCEMIA

Elevated blood sugar >200mg/dl (including random value) on antipsychotic

Abdominal symptoms, altered mental status, respiratory distress
Yes
Send for emergent evaluation
No

Pre-existing diabetes
No history of diabetes

Can tolerate acute hyperglycemia; consider urgent evaluation if blood sugar >400mg/dl with previous good control

Stop antipsychotic if previous good diabetes control

Send to primary care provider if previous poor diabetes control

Stop antipsychotic if recently initiated and monitor blood sugar

Refer to primary care provider if persistent hyperglycemia

Low threshold for urgent evaluation (e.g., mild, non-specific symptoms with any blood sugar value)

Appendix

Currently available noninsulin medication classes for diabetes mellitus

Medication class	Mechanism of action	Comments
Biguanides (metformin)	Reduces glucose production from liver and increases sensitivity to insulin	Low risk of hypoglycemia Can be used if glomerular filtration rate (GFR) >30 mL/min Vitamin B12 should be monitored periodically
Sulfonylureas (e.g., glipizide)	Increase insulin secretion	Increased risk of hypoglycemia Risk of weight gain
Dipeptidyl peptidase 4 (DDP-4) inhibitors (e.g., sitagliptin, saxagliptin)	Stimulate insulin synthesis and secretion and suppress glucagon secretion	Weight neutral Low risk for hypoglycemia
Thiazolidinediones (e.g., rosiglitazone, pioglitazone)	Reduce glucose secretion and reduce insulin resistance	Risk of weight gain Side effect of chronic edema and heart failure Increased risk of bone fractures
Glucagon-like peptide (GLP-1) agonists (e.g., liraglutide, exenatide)	Increase glucose-dependent insulin secretion	Low risk of hypoglycemia Advantage of weight loss Should not be used if history of medullary thyroid cancer Use with caution if history of pancreatitis Not orally available
Sodium glucose cotransporter 2 (SGLT-2) inhibitors (e.g., canagliflozin, empagliflozin)	Promote renal excretion of glucose	Increased risk of genital fungal infections Associated with diabetic ketoacidosis Not effective at GFR<45 mL/min
Meglitinides (e.g., repaglinide)	Increase insulin secretion	Some risk of hypoglycemia Risk of weight gain
Alpha-glucosidase inhibitors (e.g., acarbose)	Reduce postprandial glucose by preventing carbohydrate breakdown	Use limited by side effects of bloating, flatulence, diarrhea
Bile acid sequestrant (e.g., colesevelam)	May reduce intestinal glucose absorption	Use limited by side effect of constipation, dyspepsia

References

1. Mitchell AJ, Vancampfort D, Sweers K, van Winkel R, Yu W, De Hert M. Prevalence of metabolic syndrome and metabolic abnormalities in schizophrenia and related disorders--a systematic review and meta-analysis. Schizophr Bull. 2013;39(2):306–18.
2. Jin H, Meyer JM, Jeste DV. Phenomenology of and risk factors for new-onset diabetes mellitus and diabetic ketoacidosis associated with atypical antipsychotics: an analysis of 45 published cases. Ann Clin Psychiatry. 2002;14(1):59–64.

3. De Hert M, Schreurs V, Sweers K, et al. Typical and atypical antipsychotics differentially affect long-term incidence rates of the metabolic syndrome in first-episode patients with schizophrenia: a retrospective chart review. Schizophr Res. 2008;101(1-3):295–303.
4. Koller EA, Cross JT, Doraiswamy PM, Schneider BS. Risperidone-associated diabetes mellitus: a pharmacovigilance study. Pharmacotherapy. 2003;23(6):735–44.
5. Koller EA, Weber J, Doraiswamy PM, Schneider BS. A survey of reports of quetiapine-associated hyperglycemia and diabetes mellitus. J Clin Psychiatry. 2004;65(6):857–63.
6. Guenette MD, Hahn M, Cohn TA, Teo C, Remington GJ. Atypical antipsychotics and diabetic ketoacidosis: a review. Psychopharmacology (Berl). 2013;226(1):1–12.

Chapter 4
Hypertension and Acute Hypertensive Crisis

Hypertension prevalence is more than 30% in the general population and may be as high as 50% in some populations with mental illness. It is defined using cutoffs for systolic and diastolic blood pressure (SBP and DBP) that vary based on age and certain medical conditions.

An optimal blood pressure is considered to be 120/80 mmHg or less. But BP levels at which pharmacologic intervention is indicated are higher.

Pathology

Blood pressure is determined by the sympathetic nervous system, renin–angiotensin–aldosterone system and plasma volume. The majority of hypertension is primary or 'essential' and mediated by genetic and environmental factors. Risk factors to develop hypertension are advancing age, family history, obesity, physical inactivity, high sodium diet, excess alcohol intake, and presence of other cardiovascular risk factors.

Etiology

Primary hypertension is the most common reason for elevated BP. Major secondary causes are medications, alcohol, nicotine, stimulant drugs, chronic renal disease, obstructive sleep apnea, and less commonly endocrine disorders, hyperaldosteronism, pheochromocytoma.

Medications usually cause BP elevation within the normal range but sometimes can cause overt hypertension. See table for nonpsychotropic medications that can elevate BP.

© Springer International Publishing AG 2017

A. Annamalai, *Medical Management of Psychotropic Side Effects*,

DOI 10.1007/978-3-319-51026-2_4

Medications known to increase blood pressure

Oral contraceptives
Chronic nonsteroidal anti-inflammatory agent therapy
Steroids
Decongestants
Stimulants

Psychotropic Medications and Hypertension

Psychotropic agents raise BP by their effect on cholinergic, dopaminergic, and adrenergic systems. They also indirectly increase risk for hypertension by causing obesity and metabolic syndrome.

A psychotropic medication usually does not induce overt hypertension but if patient already has risk factors or a borderline high BP, the BP rise may be clinically significant.

Stimulants raise BP by 5–7 mmHg [1]. Mean BP rise with amphetamines is slightly higher than with methylphenidate. Atomoxetine causes a modest 2 mmHg BP elevation.

Among antidepressants, tricyclic antidepressants (TCAs) and serotonin norepinephrine reuptake inhibitors (SNRIs) are associated with a mean increase in blood pressure [2]. Venlafaxine causes a sustained increase in DBP; the risk is strongly dose dependent with incidence <2% at <100 mg/day and 9% at >300 mg/day [3]. Duloxetine causes a modest elevation in BP at higher doses [4]. With both medications, mean rise in BP is <10 mmHg. Bupropion, a norepinephrine dopamine reuptake inhibitor, also causes a <10 mmHg elevation in BP [1]. Monoamine oxidase inhibitors (MAOIs) rarely cause a hypertensive crisis when foods containing tyramine are ingested.

Clozapine is associated with hypertension while olanzapine is not [5]. There is uncertainty over whether the BP elevation is by a direct effect on the vasculature or indirectly through weight gain.

Mean rise in BP with psychotropic medications

Antipsychotics (clozapine)	3–5 mmHg
Antidepressants (TCAs, SNRIs, bupropion)	<10 mmHg
Stimulants (amphetamines>methylphenidate)	5–7 mmHg
Mood stabilizers (carbamazepine)	+/− (rare)

Even though the direct effect on BP from psychotropic medications is small, antipsychotic-induced weight gain can contribute to a rise in BP and metabolic syndrome. In patients with preexisting hypertension, addition of other risk factors such as obesity, diabetes, dyslipidemia worsens overall cardiovascular risk.

In the absence of coexisting factors like obesity, BP elevation from medications will reverse when the medication is stopped.

> ***Psychotropic medications usually raise BP only to a small extent and rarely induce overt hypertension.***

Clinical Features

Patients with hypertension are generally asymptomatic until they develop complications of end-organ damage, which may only occur several years after onset of illness. A significantly elevated blood pressure (considered as SBP ≥ 180 and/or DBP ≥ 120) may cause symptoms of end-organ damage like nausea/vomiting, headache, delirium, seizures, focal weakness, visual disturbance, chest pain, dyspnea, and severe back pain.

> ***Patients with hypertension are asymptomatic unless BP is very high; extreme elevations may cause symptoms of end-organ damage (e.g., headache, change in mental status, chest pain, dyspnea, focal weakness).***

Diagnosis

Hypertension should only be diagnosed after at least three separate measurements. Preferably this should be supplemented by home-based testing to eliminate predominant white coat hypertension. If there is persistent discordance between office and home measurements, 24-h ambulatory BP monitoring is recommended but this is rarely available in clinician offices. In the office, both upper arms should be alternatively used for measurement as a pressure difference >5 mmHg could signify increased risk of cardiac complications.

Previous national guidelines defined prehypertension as BP 120–139/80–89 and hypertension as 140/90 or higher. Current guidelines do not use these categories and instead define goals for therapy that are based on age and other risk factors. These are however subject to change and clinicians are encouraged to refer to the most updated Joint National Committee (JNC) guidelines.

The table lists current guidelines.

Targets for blood pressure treatment

Category	Blood pressure target (mmHg)
General population	
≥ 60 years	<150/90
<60 years	<140/90
Chronic kidney disease and diabetes	<140/90

Hypertensive urgency describes severe hypertension with no symptoms. Generally, cutoff values of SBP >180 mmHg and DBP >120 mmHg are considered severe.

Hypertensive emergency denotes severe hypertension associated with symptoms of end-organ damage.

Electrocardiogram and serum creatinine and electrolytes can identify end-organ effects from long-standing hypertension. Other tests to evaluate for organ injury with acute severe hypertension may include urinalysis, cardiac enzymes, chest radiograph, or brain imaging. A complete physical exam is also warranted to look for end-organ damage.

> ***While a BP≤120/80 mmHg is still considered optimal, threshold to initiate pharmacological treatment is higher and varies based on age and presence of chronic kidney disease or diabetes.***
>
> ***A BP >180/120 is considered severe hypertension.***

Management

Chronic Hypertension

The key to managing hypertension is prevention, as with any metabolic condition. As far as able, medications with lesser propensity to cause weight gain should be used in all patients. If a high-risk agent such as clozapine is necessary, intensive lifestyle modification should be instituted. In addition to weight loss, exercise, diet rich in vegetables and fruits, smoking cessation, limiting alcohol intake, low sodium intake all independently reduce BP. Medications that carry risk of raising BP should be avoided, if possible, in patients with unstable or untreated hypertension.

If a patient develops a rise in BP during treatment with a psychotropic agent, other immediate causes such as substance use or other offending medications should be ruled out. Regardless of the etiology, current guidelines should be followed for managing persistently high BP. Lifestyle modifications should be instituted if not already in place. Patients should be referred for long-term hypertension management if BP reaches threshold for pharmacologic treatment.

If psychotropic medication is suspected as the primary or contributing cause of elevated BP, stopping medication should be considered especially if the rise is>10 mmHg or the BP rises above the threshold for pharmacologic treatment. If BP remains high after medication is stopped due to other persistent risk factors like obesity, patient should be referred for long-term hypertension management.

Severe Hypertension

Severe hypertension without symptoms is termed hypertensive urgency. Severe hypertension with symptoms of end-organ damage is termed hypertensive emergency. Hypertensive urgency is much more likely to occur than hypertensive emergency.

Severe hypertension (BP >180/120) is unlikely to result from psychotropic medications alone.

In a patient with severe hypertension, it should be determined whether the high BP is new onset or chronic. Acute severe hypertension is more likely to result from use of illegal substance use or alcohol intoxication and withdrawal. Chronic severe hypertension is often from nonadherence to treatment or inadequate BP control with current treatment.

If severe hypertension is chronic from long-standing untreated or poorly controlled hypertension and patient is asymptomatic, then there is no medical necessity for emergent intervention. The BP can be gradually lowered over days with oral medications. If patient is already prescribed medications but is nonadherent, then pharmacotherapy should simply be restarted. If patient is on no medications, usually one agent is initiated. If patient is on a medication, a second agent is added. For gradual BP reduction, any antihypertensive is acceptable. But since treatment will be long term, medication chosen generally is one that has proven long-term cardiovascular benefit. Calcium channel blockers are a good option in patients who may not adhere to lab monitoring.

If the severe hypertension is acute, either because baseline BP is unknown or because it is significantly higher than baseline, patients should be referred for urgent evaluation even if asymptomatic. They will likely need laboratory testing and a few hours of observation to rule out any acute cardiac or neurologic event.

Patients with a known aneurysm should be referred for immediate intervention regardless of symptoms and chronicity of BP elevation. These patients, even when asymptomatic, need BP reduction over hours rather than days. And any patient with new symptoms in the setting of severe hypertension should be referred for emergent intervention regardless of whether the BP elevation is acute or chronic. They will need to be evaluated and treated for a possible cardiac or neurologic emergency.

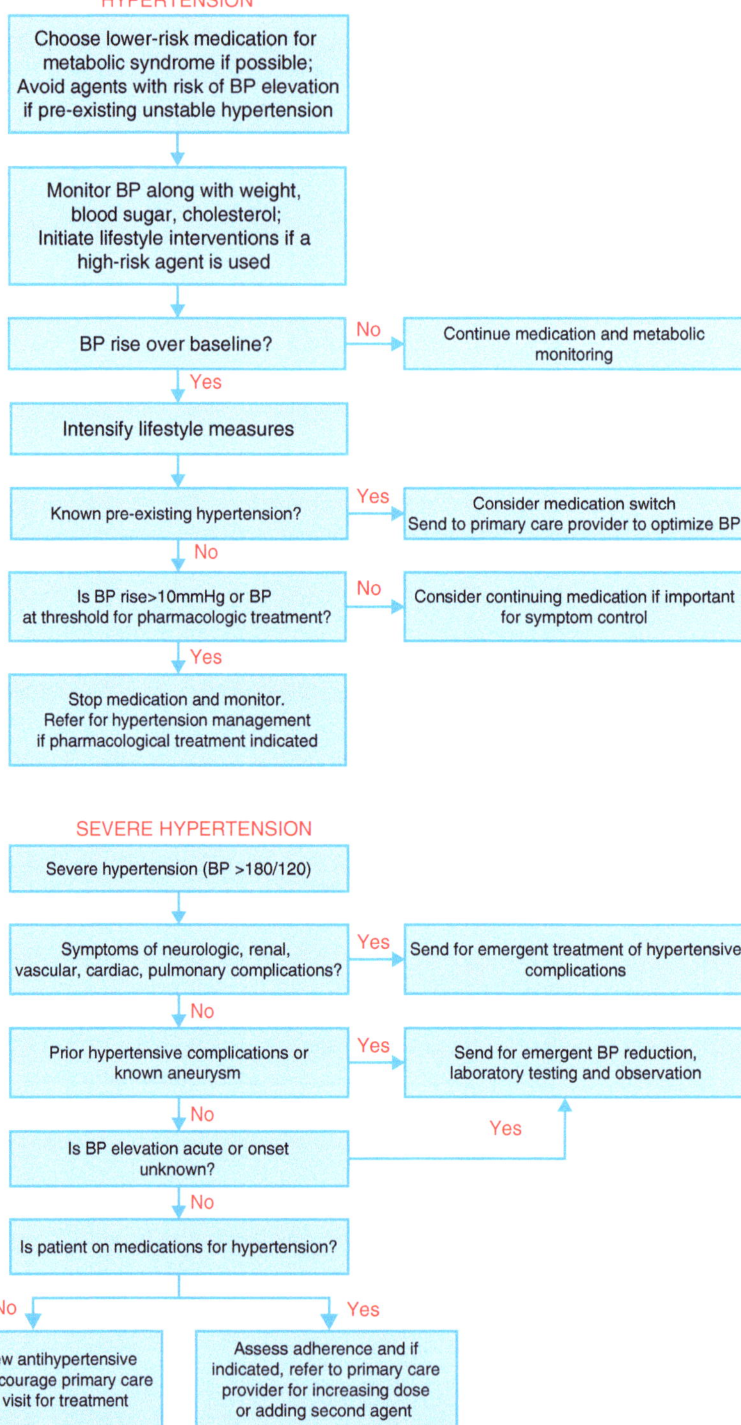
HYPERTENSION
Choose lower-risk medication for metabolic syndrome if possible; Avoid agents with risk of BP elevation if pre-existing unstable hypertension
Monitor BP along with weight, blood sugar, cholesterol; Initiate lifestyle interventions if a high-risk agent is used
BP rise over baseline?
No
Continue medication and metabolic monitoring
Yes
Intensify lifestyle measures
Known pre-existing hypertension?
Yes
Consider medication switch Send to primary care provider to optimize BP
No
Is BP rise>10mmHg or BP at threshold for pharmacologic treatment?
No
Consider continuing medication if important for symptom control
Yes
Stop medication and monitor. Refer for hypertension management if pharmacological treatment indicated
SEVERE HYPERTENSION
Severe hypertension (BP >180/120)
Symptoms of neurologic, renal, vascular, cardiac, pulmonary complications?
Yes
Send for emergent treatment of hypertensive complications
No
Prior hypertensive complications or known aneurysm
Yes
Send for emergent BP reduction, laboratory testing and observation
No
Yes
Is BP elevation acute or onset unknown?
No
Is patient on medications for hypertension?
No
Yes
Initiate new antihypertensive agent or encourage primary care provider visit for treatment
Assess adherence and if indicated, refer to primary care provider for increasing dose or adding second agent

Appendix

Guidelines from Joint National Commission (JNC-8) [6]

Thiazide diuretics, calcium channel blockers (CCBs), angiotensin-converting enzyme inhibitors (ACEIs), or angiotensin receptor blockers (ARBs) are all considered first-line medications for hypertension treatment

For black patients, including those with diabetes, CCBs or thiazide diuretics should be first-line medications

For all patients with chronic kidney disease, regardless of race or diabetes status, ACEIs or ARBs should be included in antihypertensive treatment

Beta blockers should only be considered after thiazine diuretics, CCBs, ACEIs, ARBs, unless other indications like ischemic heart disease or heart failure are present

If BP is not at goal after 1 month on medication, dose should be raised or second agent added; medications should be added until goal BP is reached

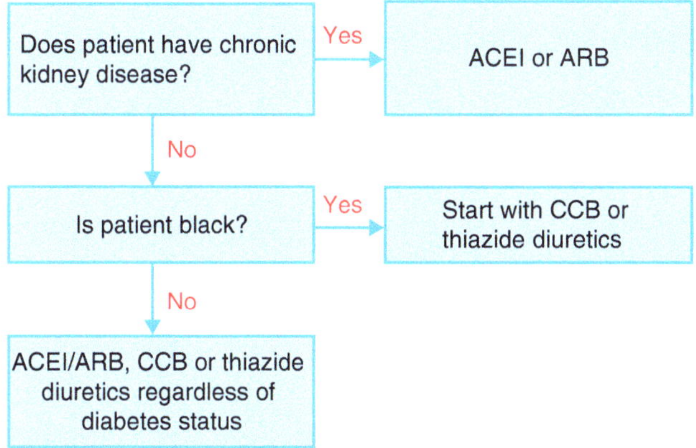

Commonly used medications for hypertension

Medication class	Mechanism of action	Comments
Thiazide diuretics Hydrochlorothiazide Chlorthalidone	Inhibit sodium transport in the distal renal tubule	Serum potassium should be monitored
ACEI Lisinopril Enalapril Captopril	Inhibit conversion of angiotensin I to II resulting in vasodilation and reduced sympathetic activity	Renal function and serum potassium should be monitored
ARB Losartan Candesartan Valsartan	Block angiotensin II receptors in blood vessels resulting in vasodilation and reduced sympathetic activity	Generally only indicated if ACEIs are not tolerated (e.g., cough occurs with ACEIs and not ARBs)

(continued)

(continued)

Medication class	Mechanism of action	Comments
CCBs *Dihydropyridine* Amlodipine *Nondihydropyridine* Verapamil Diltiazem	Regulate calcium influx into vascular smooth muscle cells and reduce vascular resistance	No lab monitoring required Nondihydropyridines generally used only with additional indications (e.g., atrial fibrillation)
Beta blockers Metoprolol Atenolol Carvedilol	Block beta receptors in blood vessels and reduce sympathetic tone	Not used unless additional indications (e.g., atrial fibrillation, angina, heart failure) and first-line agents already used Metoprolol and atenolol are cardioselective and preferred in obstructive lung disease

References

1. Wilens TE, Hammerness PG, Biederman J, Kwon A, Spencer TJ, Clark S, et al. Blood pressure changes associated with medication treatment of adults with attention-deficit/hyperactivity disorder. J Clin Psychiatry. 2005;66(2):253–9.
2. Licht CM, de Geus EJ, Seldenrijk A, van Hout HP, Zitman FG, van Dyck R, et al. Depression is associated with decreased blood pressure, but antidepressant use increases the risk for hypertension. Hypertension. 2009;53(4):631–8.
3. Thase ME. Effects of venlafaxine on blood pressure: a meta-analysis of original data from 3744 depressed patients. J Clin Psychiatry. 1998;59(10):502–8.
4. Thase ME, Tran PV, Wiltse C, Pangallo BA, Mallinckrodt C, Detke MJ. Cardiovascular profile of duloxetine, a dual reuptake inhibitor of serotonin and norepinephrine. J Clin Psychopharmacol. 2005;25(2):132–40.
5. Woo YS, Kim W, Chae JH, Yoon BH, Bahk WM. Blood pressure changes during clozapine or olanzapine treatment in Korean schizophrenic patients. World J Biol Psychiatry. 2009; 10(4 Pt 2):420–5.
6. James PA, Oparil S, Carter BL, Cushman WC, Dennison-Himmelfarb C, Handler J, et al. Evidence-based guideline for the management of high blood pressure in adults: report from the panel members appointed to the Eighth Joint National Committee (JNC 8). JAMA. 2014;311(5):507–20.

Chapter 5
Hyperlipidemia

Hyperlipidemia is an abnormality in lipid levels. It is commonly described as one or more of the following: high total cholesterol (TC), high low-density lipoprotein cholesterol (LDL-C), high triglycerides (TG), low high-density lipoprotein cholesterol (HDL-C).

Optimal values for these lipids are based on individual risk factors.

Pathology

Lipids are of concern mainly due to their association with atherosclerosis and increased risk of cardiovascular events. Lipids such as cholesterol and TGs are transported by lipoproteins to various tissues. In addition to HDL and LDL, other lipoproteins include chylomicrons, very low-density lipoprotein (VLDL), and intermediate-density lipoprotein (IDL). They each carry varying degrees of cholesterol and TGs, with LDL-C carrying the majority of cholesterol and VLDL and chylomicrons carrying the majority of TGs.

A standard serum lipid profile measures TC, HDL-C, and TGs; LDL-C is generally calculated though it can be measured directly. The LDL-C calculation is affected by the amount of triglycerides in the blood, which is higher in the nonfasting state. TC and HDL-C, which are directly measured, do not differ significantly in the nonfasting state.

Cholesterol levels are directly related to cardiovascular risk by accelerating atherosclerosis. TGs are also associated with elevated cardiovascular risk but it is not clear if the relationship is causal.

HDL-C removes cholesterol from cells of arterial walls and is associated with decreased atherosclerosis. Hence, higher levels are associated with lower cardiovascular risk.

© Springer International Publishing AG 2017

A. Annamalai, *Medical Management of Psychotropic Side Effects*,

DOI 10.1007/978-3-319-51026-2_5

Etiology

Disorders in lipid metabolism can occur from genetic mutations that affect either production or clearance of lipoproteins resulting in elevated TGs and cholesterol. But secondary causes are more common reasons for dyslipidemia. Common secondary etiologies are sedentary lifestyle, excess dietary intake of cholesterol, and obesity. Other secondary etiologies are diabetes mellitus, chronic kidney disease, hypothyroidism, cholestatic liver disease, and certain medications.

Psychotropic Medications and Lipid Disorders

Antipsychotics with increased propensity for metabolic syndrome also increase risk for developing lipid disorders. The mechanism is mainly via increased weight and resulting insulin resistance. There may also be adiposity-independent effects on glucose and lipid metabolism [1] though no receptor targets have been identified as causative. Increases in TGs and TC have been seen as early as 4 months after antipsychotic initiation [2]. Similar to metabolic syndrome, clozapine and olanzapine carry the highest risk of dyslipidemia while ziprasidone and aripiprazole carry the least risk.

Olanzapine and other antipsychotics are also associated with severe hypertriglyceridemia that is independent of and occurs before weight gain is established. The mechanism is hypothesized to be due to a direct effect on triglyceride metabolism and indirect effect on inflammation and insulin resistance [3]. As with obesity and other metabolic side effects, propensity to cause hypertriglyceridemia is highest with olanzapine and clozapine. Extreme elevations of triglycerides can cause pancreatitis and hypertriglyceridemia may be the mechanism in at least some cases of pancreatitis induced by clozapine and olanzapine.

Statins and other agents that are effective in improving lipid profile in the general population are also effective in people on antipsychotics. When the offending medication is stopped, the lipid abnormalities may reverse if weight reduces. Acute elevation in triglycerides has been documented to improve when the medication is stopped.

Antidepressants also may adversely affect lipid profile and the mechanism is thought to be predominantly due to weight increase from medications that promote weight gain [4]. Among mood stabilizers, carbamazepine may increase lipids while valproate and lithium do not [5].

> *Antipsychotic-induced hyperlipidemia occurs mostly related to weight gain; however, there may be weight-independent lipid abnormalities, especially hypertriglyceridemia that occurs early in treatment.*

Clinical Features

Hyperlipidemia is generally asymptomatic until it causes complications like coronary artery disease or stroke or triglyceride pancreatitis. But high levels can cause xanthomas that are firm and nontender skin deposits of cholesterol-rich cells in tendons, joint surfaces, hands, and feet.

> ***Hyperlipidemia is much more likely to be diagnosed by lab testing than by signs or symptoms.***

Diagnosis

Hyperlipidemia is diagnosed by direct measurement of TC, HDL-C, TGs, and calculation of LDL-C. Non-HDL cholesterol is more predictive of cardiovascular risk than LDL-C and can be calculated (Non-HDL-C = TC−HDL-C).

Lipid profile does not need to be measured in a fasting state. The TC and HDL-C, which are used to predict cardiovascular risk, vary only slightly between fasting and nonfasting states. But a fasting state is required for accurate TG measurement. LDL-C calculation depends on fasting TG levels but it can be directly measured in a nonfasting state.

Since treatment decisions for lipid abnormalities are based on cardiovascular risk, the threshold for treatment depends on other risk factors. Cardiovascular risk calculators are available to estimate risk for individuals. While none is the gold standard and applicable to all populations, a commonly used one is the tool used by American Heart Association and American College of Cardiology AHA/ACC Pooled Cohort Equations CV Risk Calculator (http://clincalc.com/Cardiology/ASCVD/PooledCohort.aspx).

Current guidelines provide thresholds for pharmacologic treatment as shown in the table. However, these guidelines are subject to change and readers are encouraged to refer to the latest recommendations by AHA and ACC.

Criteria for treatment with statins
• Individuals with clinical atherosclerotic cardiovascular disease (ASCVD)
• Individuals with primary elevations of LDL-C ≥190 mg/dL
• Individuals 40 to 75 years of age with diabetes and without ASCVD and LDL-C 70 to 189 mg/dL
• Individuals 40 to 75 years of age without clinical ASCVD or diabetes and LDL-C 70 to 189 mg/dL and a 10-year ASCVD risk of 7.5% or higher

Serum triglycerides >150 mg/dL is considered high and values >500 mg/dL generally need pharmacological intervention.

> ***Determining treatment thresholds for serum lipids depends on other cardiovascular risk factors; elevated triglyceride levels independently predict risk of pancreatitis.***

Management

As with other conditions that are part of metabolic syndrome, prevention is the best treatment for dyslipidemia. Medications that are less likely to cause weight gain and lipid abnormalities should be used whenever possible. Lifestyle modification is similar to what is recommended for obesity. They should be aggressively instituted for patients who need to be on high-risk medications such as clozapine.

Lipids should be measured in 3 months after starting an antipsychotic. If weight and lipids remain stable after 6 months of treatment, lipids can be measured yearly. More frequent measurements will be needed if there is initial elevation of lipids. If lipid abnormalities develop during antipsychotic treatment, other easily identifiable causes such as thyroid disorders, kidney or liver disease, diabetes mellitus, and medications like steroids or estrogens should be screened for.

As with any metabolic disorder, the offending medication should be stopped, if possible, to halt or possibly reverse the weight gain and lipid abnormalities. Pharmacologic treatment for lipid abnormalities is similar to treatment of hyperlipidemia that is not induced by medications. Statins are the mainstay of treatment for treating hyperlipidemia and reducing cardiovascular risk.

The Appendix lists statin recommendations for different cardiovascular risk categories.

Acute Hypertriglyceridemia

Generally, a TG level >150 mg/dL requires modification of diet and exercise, similar to treatment of obesity. There is some correlation between elevated TG levels and cardiovascular risk. Treatment with statins at lower TG levels is sufficient for overall cardiovascular risk reduction. If the TG rises >500 mg/dL, medications to specifically target TG are warranted. At moderate to high TG levels there is a risk for acute pancreatitis. The average serum TG level in people with TG-induced pancreatitis is >2000 mg/dL. But even a TG>1000 mg/dL should be considered a risk for pancreatitis especially in people with history of past episodes. Fibrates are effective pharmacologic agents for lowering TG.

If an elevation in triglycerides occurs after initiation of an atypical antipsychotic, the medication should be stopped if possible. If the medication is necessary, then the TG should be closely monitored. If the level rises >500 mg/dL, patient should be referred for treatment with fibrates. If pancreatitis occurs, it is recommended not to reinitiate the causative agent.

People with known alcohol use are at higher risk of pancreatitis and this should be an additional consideration when selecting antipsychotics that also increase the risk of hypertriglyceridemia and pancreatitis.

Medication switch and structured lifestyle interventions are recommended initial interventions if hyperlipidemia occurs on antipsychotic medication.

Statins are used for cardiovascular risk reduction and fibrates to reduce triglyceride levels and risk of pancreatitis.

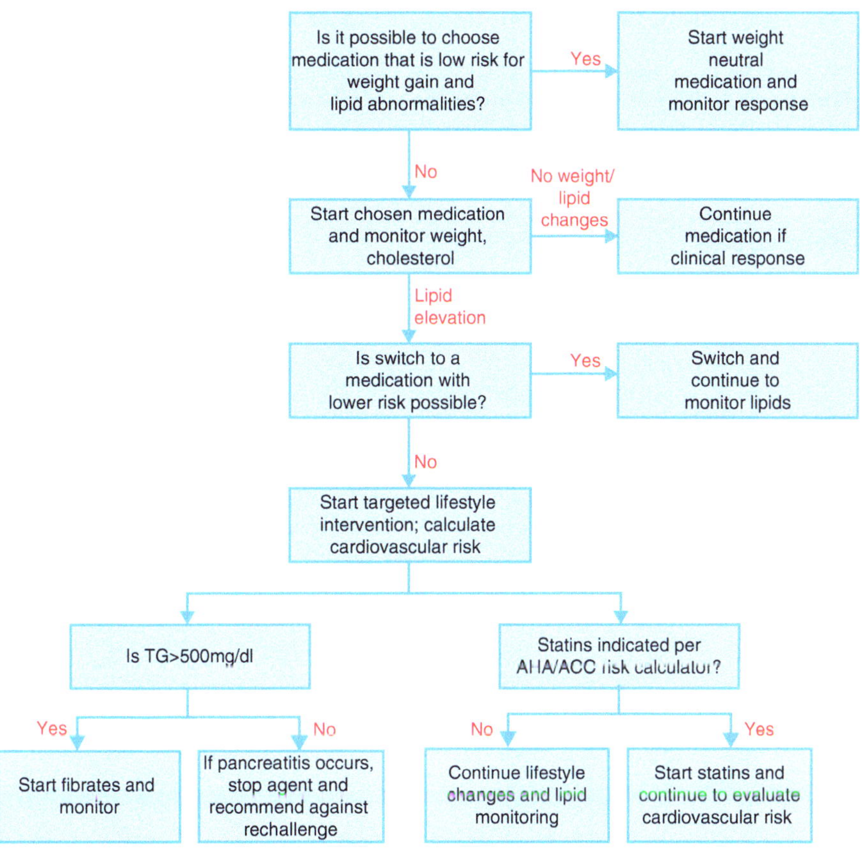

Appendix

Clinical characteristic	Statin intensity
Clinical ASCVD (Age >21)	High[a]
Serum LDL > 190 mg/dL *OR* non-HDL > 220 mg/dL (Age >21)	High
Diabetes (Age 40–75)	Moderate to high
10-year risk greater than 7.5% (Age 40–75)	Moderate[b]

[a]High-Intensity Statins Therapy (~50% cholesterol reduction): Atorvastatin 80 mg (40 mg less preferred), Rosuvastatin 20–40 mg

[b]Moderate-Intensity Statin Therapy (30–50% cholesterol reduction): Atorvastatin 10–20 mg, Rosuvastatin 5–10 mg, Simvastatin 20–40 mg, Pravastatin 40–80 mg, Lovastatin 40 mg, Fluvastatin 80 mg (80 mg XL daily or 40 mg BID), Pitavastatin 2–4 mg

References

1. Newcomer JW. Antipsychotic medications: metabolic and cardiovascular risk. J Clin Psychiatry. 2007;68(Suppl 4):8–13.
2. Tse L, Procyshyn RM, Fredrikson DH, Boyda HN, Honer WG, Barr AM. Pharmacological treatment of antipsychotic-induced dyslipidemia and hypertension. Int Clin Psychopharmacol. 2014;29(3):125–37.
3. Yan H, Chen JD, Zheng XY. Potential mechanisms of atypical antipsychotic-induced hypertriglyceridemia. Psychopharmacology (Berl). 2013;229(1):1–7.
4. McIntyre RS, Soczynska JK, Konarski JZ, Kennedy SH. The effect of antidepressants on lipid homeostasis: a cardiac safety concern? Expert Opin Drug Saf. 2006;5(4):523–37.
5. Sonmez FM, Demir E, Orem A, et al. Effect of antiepileptic drugs on plasma lipids, lipoprotein (a), and liver enzymes. J Child Neurol. 2006;21(1):70–4.

Section III
Cardiovascular System

Chapter 6
Orthostatic Hypotension

Orthostatic hypotension is the fall in arterial blood pressure (BP) in the upright posture due to loss of vasoconstrictor reflexes in lower extremity blood vessels. It is defined as >20 mmHg fall in systolic blood pressure (SBP) and >10 mmHg fall in diastolic blood pressure (DBP). It is more common in the elderly, especially with antihypertensive treatment. Prevalence is as high as 20% in people over age 65.

Pathology

The normal vascular response with assumption of the upright posture is pooling of blood in lower extremities → decreased venous return to the heart → reduced cardiac output → compensatory increase in sympathetic outflow → increased peripheral resistance, venous return, cardiac output → limit the fall in BP to 5–10 mmHg SBP.

A disruption in the compensatory mechanism results in a greater fall in BP when the body assumes an upright posture.

Etiology

Orthostatic hypotension is caused by disease conditions that impair autonomic reflexes resulting in a failure to increase peripheral resistance and venous return to the heart. It can also occur when there is significant intravascular volume depletion. Medications cause orthostatic hypotension by multiple mechanisms including vasodilation, volume depletion, and autonomic dysfunction. Major etiologies are listed in the table.

© Springer International Publishing AG 2017

A. Annamalai, *Medical Management of Psychotropic Side Effects*,

DOI 10.1007/978-3-319-51026-2_6

Common etiologies for orthostatic hypotension

Vasovagal reflex
Prolonged best rest
Primary autonomic dysfunction (e.g., Parkinson disease)
Peripheral neuropathy (e.g., diabetes, alcohol)
Volume depletion (e.g., diarrhea)
Postprandial hypotension
Congestive heart failure
Medications (e.g., antihypertensives, vasodilators, diuretics, sedatives, opiates, antipsychotics, antidepressants)

Psychotropic Medications and Orthostatic Hypotension

Orthostatic hypotension is a common side effect of antipsychotics and causes syncope in a small proportion of patients. Both the hypotension and syncope are most commonly reported with clozapine [1]. It is thought to result mainly from blockade of alpha-1 receptors in peripheral blood vessels thus interfering with the vasoconstrictor response to peripheral pooling of blood. Other mechanisms are vasodilation from cholinergic blockade and central effect on autonomic regulation and baroreceptor reflexes [2]. In general, lower potency agents are more likely to cause orthostatic hypotension. The hypotension occurs early in treatment and often patients develop tolerance to this side effect. It is reversible on stopping the offending medication.

Among antidepressants, tricyclic antidepressants (TCAs) and older monoamine oxidase inhibitors (MAOIs) can cause orthostatic hypotension by alpha-adrenergic blockade. Selective serotonergic reuptake inhibitors (SSRIs) are only rarely associated with orthostatic hypotension [3]. Mirtazapine has moderate alpha-adrenergic blockade and occasionally causes orthostatic hypotension. Trazodone is also associated with this side effect. Wellbutrin is not associated with orthostatic hypotension.

Mood stabilizers are not associated with orthostatic hypotension.

Risk factors for developing orthostatic hypotension include polypharmacy, older age, preexisting cardiac, or metabolic disease.

Psychotropic medications causing orthostatic hypotension (decreasing order of likelihood)

Antipsychotics
Clozapine, chlorpromazine
Quetiapine, risperidone, iloperidone,
Perphenazine, olanzapine, ziprasidone, lurasidone, aripiprazole
Antidepressants
TCAs, MAOIs
Trazodone
Mirtazapine

Antipsychotics are commonly associated with orthostatic hypotension, increasing risk of syncope. It occurs early in treatment and tolerance often develops to this effect.

Clinical Features

Patient may complain of symptoms of dizziness, clamminess, sweating with change in position, and generalized fatigue. In more severe cases, there may be falls, visual disturbance, or transient loss of consciousness. Palpitations and tachycardia may be present.

Patients will commonly complain of light-headedness especially with change in position. Falls can occur when symptoms are severe.

Diagnosis

BP and heart rate (HR) should be measured in supine and standing positions with at least 2 min between positions. Patient can be sitting if unable to stand. A fall in BP as described earlier is usually accompanied by an increase HR >15 beats/min. If a primary autonomic failure is present, then this compensatory rise in HR may not be seen.

In patients who develop orthostatic hypotension due to a psychotropic medication, the timing of symptoms establishes the diagnosis. But other etiologies like volume depletion, nonpsychotropic medications, worsening diabetes, and cardiac disease should be ruled out.

Blood pressure should be measured in supine position and then standing or sitting, at least two minutes apart to accurately assess for an orthostatic drop; if this is infeasible, a clear report of positional symptoms may suffice to inform management.

Management

As far as possible, patients with preexisting risk factors (including treatment with multiple antihypertensives) for developing orthostatic hypotension should be started on psychotropic agents that are less likely to cause this side effect. If such a medication is necessary, then dose titration should occur slowly. If the side effect does develop, patients should be evaluated for other precipitating and contributing factors. Reason for treating the orthostatic hypotension is generally for disabling symptoms. If symptoms are mild, the offending medication can still be continued unless baseline BP is low. Tolerance may develop to orthostatic hypotension that results from a medication.

If tolerance does not develop and patient remains symptomatic, some simple measures may help reduce symptoms. See table for some recommendations. If non-pharmacological measures are inadequate, medications are available to treat this side effect. It is rare to utilize these for orthostatic hypotension resulting from psychotropic use. An example where this might be necessary is clozapine, which may be difficult to discontinue. Medications that have been used with clozapine to treat orthostatic hypotension are fludrocortisone (a mineralocorticoid that acts by increasing sodium retention) and ephedrine (an alpha-adrenergic agonist) [4].

Recommended nonpharmacological measures to reduce orthostatic hypotension

Avoid abrupt changes in posture
Sit for a few minutes before standing upon waking in the morning
Increase fluid intake
Avoid heat and dehydration
Increase salt intake (if no hypertension, cardiac, or kidney disease)
Avoid straining during micturition and defecation, if possible
Limit alcohol use
Physical maneuvers upon standing—tensing legs by crossing legs, hand grip by clenching fist over an object
Support stockings that are waist high (generally not well tolerated by patients)

> *Psychotropic medication can be continued for mild tolerable orthostatic symptoms.*
>
> *Nonpharmacological measures are often sufficient in symptomatic orthostatic hypotension.*
>
> *Adjunctive medications can be considered in clozapine-induced orthostatic hypotension.*

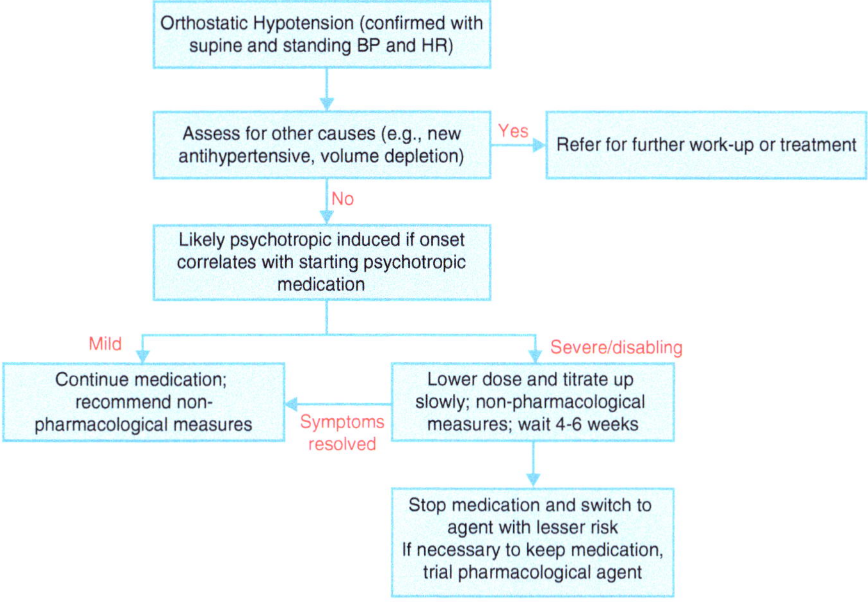

References

1. Mackin P. Cardiac side effects of psychiatric drugs. Hum Psychopharmacol. 2008;23(Suppl 1): 3–14.
2. Leung JY, Barr AM, Procyshyn RM, Honer WG, Pang CC. Cardiovascular side-effects of anti-psychotic drugs: the role of the autonomic nervous system. Pharmacol Ther. 2012;135(2): 113–22.
3. Pacher P, Kecskemeti V. Cardiovascular side effects of new antidepressants and antipsychotics: new drugs, old concerns? Curr Pharm Des. 2004;10(20):2463–75.
4. Young CR, Bowers Jr MB, Mazure CM. Management of the adverse effects of clozapine. Schizophr Bull. 1998;24(3):381–90.

Chapter 7
Tachycardia and Myocarditis

Tachyarrhythmias are defined as rhythms with a heart rate >100 beats/min. Sinus tachycardia is a fast but regular rhythm.

Pathology

Sinus tachycardia is due to an increase in cardiac impulses arising in the sino-atrial node. It is almost always due to a secondary cause, either cardiac disease or systemic illness. Long-standing severe tachycardia may be deleterious to cardiac function due to reduction of cardiac output and reduced coronary blood flow.

Etiology

The following table lists common conditions resulting in sinus tachycardia.

Conditions resulting in sinus tachycardia

Volume depletion
Hypotension
Systemic infections/fever
Pain
Anxiety
Stimulant use
Withdrawal of beta-blockers
Acute coronary disease and heart failure
Acute and chronic pulmonary disease
Hyperthyroidism

© Springer International Publishing AG 2017

A. Annamalai, *Medical Management of Psychotropic Side Effects*,

DOI 10.1007/978-3-319-51026-2_7

Psychotropic Medications and Tachycardia

All antipsychotics cause some degree of tachycardia, mainly due to cardiac cholinergic blockade. Clozapine with the strongest relative affinity for this receptor can cause more than a 20% increase in heart rate. Even so, this is rarely clinically relevant. Slow titration of clozapine may prevent development of tachycardia. If the tachycardia is treated, it responds to beta blockers and calcium channel blockers. The tachycardia resolves if clozapine is stopped.

The possibility of myocarditis with clozapine should be considered when tachycardia occurs. Tachycardia with clozapine is common while myocarditis is rare. Both develop in the first few days to weeks of medication initiation. Clozapine is also associated with cardiomyopathy [1] and this may be related to acute myocarditis or due to tachycardia-mediated ventricular dysfunction. Generally, if tachycardia is the only presentation, there is no need for evaluation for myocarditis or cardiomyopathy. See table for clinical and diagnostic features of clozapine-induced myocarditis. Symptoms of cardiomyopathy such as dyspnea and fatigue may develop more insidiously if it occurs without preceding myocarditis.

Clozapine-induced myocarditis

It is an immune-mediated hypersensitivity reaction to medication
Pathology: Eosinophilic infiltration in myocardial cells
Other causes: Other medications, viral, idiopathic
Onset: Incidence is 1% and most occur within 2 weeks of clozapine initiation
Signs and symptoms: Tachycardia, fever, chest pain, dyspnea, hypotension, or other signs of heart failure
Diagnosis:
EKG: Nonspecific ST-T changes, arrhythmias
Serum tests: Elevated cardiac biomarkers, eosinophilia, high c-reactive protein, or erythrocyte sedimentation rate
Echocardiogram: Decreased ejection fraction if cardiomyopathy present
Cardiac magnetic resonance: Increased myocardial signaling
Endomyocardial biopsy (gold standard but not typically done): Eosinophilic infiltration
Management: Stop clozapine immediately; treatment of cardiac arrhythmias and ventricular dysfunction
Clozapine rechallenge is not recommended

Tricyclic antidepressants also cause some tachycardia due to a basal increase in serum norepinephrine. Stimulant medications can also increase heart rate but the increase is small and generally not clinically concerning.

Clozapine may cause 20% rise in heart rate but is rarely clinically significant; if any other systemic symptoms, myocarditis should be considered.

Clinical Features

Tachycardia alone usually does not cause symptoms. But if tachycardia is severe, patients may experience palpitations. Symptomatic tachycardia can rarely lead to angina or dyspnea due to its effects on cardiac functioning.

Tachycardia is usually asymptomatic unless severe.

Diagnosis

Sinus tachycardia is readily identifiable on an EKG as a fast sinus rhythm. P waves are clearly identifiable, each P wave is followed by a QRS complex, and the RR intervals are uniform. Generally the heart rate is <140 beats/min. At higher heart rates >140 beats/min, sinus tachycardia is less easily distinguished from other tachyarrhythmias arising from outside the sinus node.

The EKG changes of acute myocarditis are nonspecific. Changes related to cardiomyopathy may resemble those of cardiac ischemia. Echocardiogram and cardiac magnetic resonance imaging are necessary when these conditions are suspected.

Following is a rhythm strip showing sinus tachycardia around 100 beats/min.

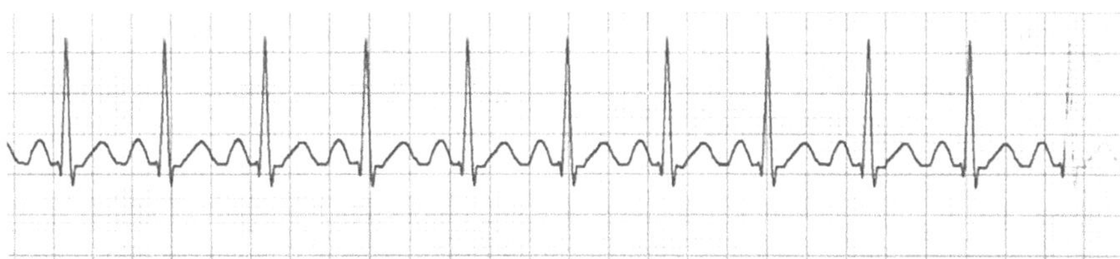

If every P wave is followed by a QRS complex and the RR intervals are equal the rhythm is sinus; generally heart rate is <140 beats/min for sinus tachycardia.

Management

If baseline heart rate is high, it should be evaluated and treated appropriately before initiating antipsychotics, especially clozapine since it can worsen the tachycardia. Tachycardia on treatment, regardless of the extent, is not a reason to discontinue the psychotropic agent in the absence of cardiac complications. However, clinicians should remember that it can worsen underlying cardiac symptoms in those with preexisting unstable coronary artery disease or cardiac failure and this is one factor to consider when initiating medications that cause significant tachycardia.

In general, patients on clozapine do not have a heart rate>120 beats/min and there is no need to treat the tachycardia if asymptomatic. There is no specific cutoff for when to treat the tachycardia. Medications to treat tachycardia from clozapine is recommended if patient develops symptoms or preexisting cardiac disease make long-term complications more likely. Medications successfully tried in case reports are beta blockers (atenolol, propranolol), calcium channel blockers (verapamil), and ivabradine (a cardiac agent used to slow heart rate in heart failure) [2].

Tachycardia is usually not a reason to discontinue medication.

If clozapine-induced tachycardia is >120 beats/min, associated with symptoms or complicates underlying cardiac disease, atenolol, propranolol, or verapamil can be considered as first-line treatment.

If any additional cardiac symptoms occur, myocarditis and cardiomyopathy should be considered.

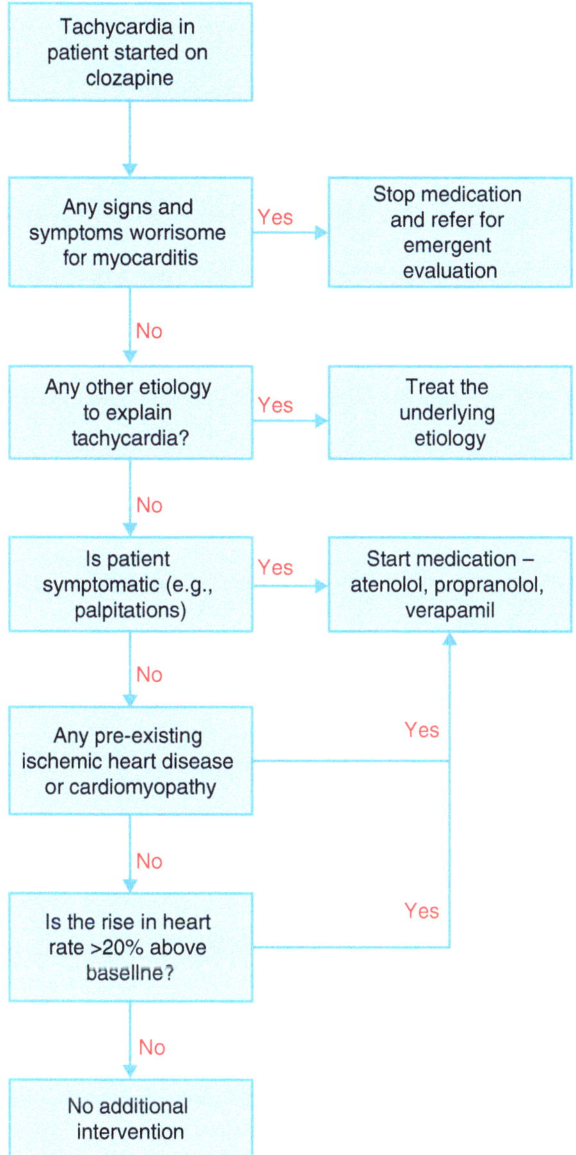

References

1. La Grenade L, Graham D, Trontell A. Myocarditis and cardiomyopathy associated with clozapine use in the United States. N Engl J Med. 2001;345(3):224–5.
2. Lally J, Docherty MJ, MacCabe JH. Pharmacological interventions for clozapine-induced sinus tachycardia. Cochrane Database Syst Rev. 2016;6:CD011566.

Chapter 8
QTc Prolongation

The EKG waveform starts with the P wave, which represents atrial depolarization and ends with the T wave, which represents the end of ventricular repolarization.

The QT interval on an electrocardiogram (EKG) represents ventricular depolarization and repolarization. QTc is a corrected interval that corrects for influence of heart rate on the QT interval. QT prolongation increases the risk of torsades pointes, a potentially fatal arrhythmia and it has thus become a surrogate marker for drug-related cardiac complications.

A QTc <440 ms is considered normal in males and a QTc <450 ms is considered normal in females.

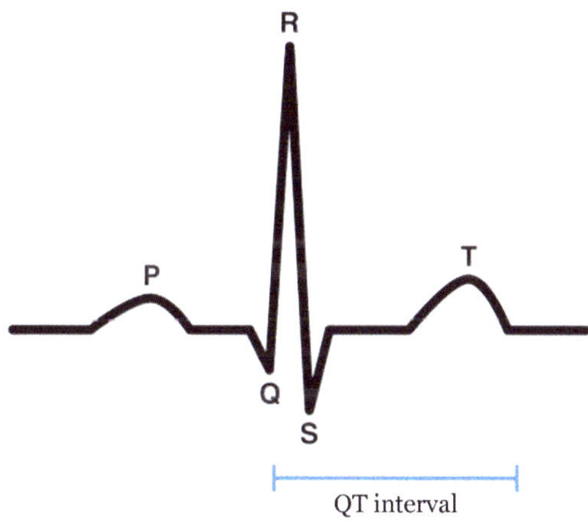

QTc is the interval from the beginning of the Q wave to the end of the T wave.

Normal values are <440 ms in males and <450 ms in females.

© Springer International Publishing AG 2017
A. Annamalai, *Medical Management of Psychotropic Side Effects*,
DOI 10.1007/978-3-319-51026-2_8

Pathology

Acquired QTc prolongation is mostly drug induced. The common mechanism is formation of early after depolarization and prolonged repolarization by blockade of ion channels in cardiac cells. The after depolarization can trigger an arrhythmia and increase risk for torsades de pointes (TdP), a form of polymorphic ventricular tachycardia occurring in the setting of a prolonged QTc interval. The term, meaning "twisting of the points," refers to the pattern of the polymorphic ventricular tachycardia seen on the EKG.

QTc prolongation is related to the risk of cardiac mortality, presumably by causing TdP. However, the extent of medication-induced QTc prolongation does not always correlate with level of TdP risk.

> *QTc prolongation is a risk factor for TdP, a malignant ventricular arrhythmia, but the risk of Tdp with a medication is not always directly proportional to its risk of QTc prolongation.*

Etiology

Most QTc prolongation is acquired. Medications and electrolyte abnormalities are the most common causes. Medical conditions that increase risk of electrolyte imbalance, predispose to other arrhythmias, or interfere in metabolism of QTc prolonging medications increase risk of QTc prolongation.

See table for risk factors and conditions associated with QTc prolongation. A complete list of medications that can prolong QTc can be found at www.crediblemeds.org.

Causes and risk factors for prolonged QTc [1]

Female gender
Increased age
Congenital QT syndrome
Electrolyte abnormalities (hypokalemia, hypocalcemia, hypomagnesemia)
Cardiac conditions (bradycardia, left ventricular dysfunction, heart failure, mitral valve prolapse, myocardial infarction)
Conditions that affect electrolyte balance (anorexia nervosa, malnutrition, obesity)
Chronic medical conditions (renal and hepatic dysfunction, hypothyroidism, central nervous system injury, diabetes, hypertension, acquired immune deficiency syndrome)
Nonpsychotropic medications (class I&III antiarrhythmics, macrolide and quinolone antibiotics, azole antifungals, furosemide, tamoxifen)

Psychotropic Medications and QTc

Psychotropic medications prolong QTc by binding to cardiac potassium channels. The QTc prolongation increases the risk of cardiac arrhythmia and sudden death but the absolute risk with these agents remains small. The QTc prolongation can occur at any dose but the risk increases with dose.

Among antipsychotics, ziprasidone causes a greater QT prolongation than many other agents but the absolute increase is modest. It increases QTc >60 ms in <1% of patients and it is rare to see QTc >500 ms (0.06%) [1]. Very few case reports have described TdP with ziprasidone and sudden death has been associated with ziprasidone in less than ten cases [2]. The overall risk of sudden death with ziprasidone is no higher than with comparator medications [3]. Though QTc prolongation is generally dose dependent, the effect with ziprasidone does not seem to depend on dose.

Low-potency antipsychotics are thought to have a higher risk of prolonging QTc, though haloperidol is an exception. Haloperidol prolongs QTc to a lesser extent than ziprasidone but is associated with a higher risk of TdP. Intravenous haloperidol carries a higher risk of TdP than oral or intramuscular administration.

There is some information on newer antipsychotics [4]. Iloperidone may cause QTc prolongation comparable to ziprasidone [5]. Paliperidone causes some QTc prolongation [6] while lurasidone does not appear to cause QTc prolongation.

Among antidepressants, citalopram is the only agent to which the Food and Drug Administration (FDA) attached a warning label [7]. The FDA recommends against doses >40 mg. There is only a modest increase in QTc at 60 mg but the additional clinical benefit is not considered significant enough to warrant an additional risk. There are also case reports of TdP with citalopram. It is unclear whether the overall mortality from citalopram is higher at >40 mg/day but the FDA warning label will remain until further evidence becomes available. Escitalopram increases QTc to a much lesser extent and the FDA has placed no restrictions on its use. No other serotonin reuptake inhibitors have a clinically significant effect on QTc. Tricyclic antidepressants prolong QTc mainly by widening the QRS interval.

Among mood stabilizers, lithium at high doses can increase the QTc but is not associated with TdP. Methadone can increase QTc and is a cause for TdP. Antihistamines have a small risk of QTc prolongation.

See the following tables for QTc prolongation with different psychotropic medications.

QTc prolongation risk with psychotropic agents

High risk	Thioridazine, pimozide, intravenous haloperidol, ziprasidone (but less association with torsades), citalopram
Moderate risk	Chlorpromazine, fluphenazine, oral/intramuscular haloperidol (less risk than intravenous but associated with TdP), iloperidone, risperdione, escitalopram, tricyclic antidepressants
Low risk	Asenapine, lurasidone, olanzapine, quetiapine, paliperidone
Minimal risk	Aripiprazole, clozapine

Mean QTc change in milliseconds

• Aripiprazole—0
• Clozapine—0
• Olanzapine—0–6
• Risperidone—0–11
• Quetiapine—0–14
• Haloperidol (oral) —4–7
• Escitalopram—4.5/10.7 (10 mg/30 mg)
• Citalopram—8.5/12.6/18.5 (20 mg/40 mg/60 mg)
• Pimozide—13
• Ziprasidone—4–22
• Thioridazine—25–30

> *The absolute risk of QTc prolongation and TdP with psychotropic agents is small.*
>
> *Ziprasidone causes more QTc prolongation but carries less risk of TdP than haloperidol.*

Clinical Features

Palpitations, dizziness, or syncopal attacks may be warning signs of episodes of TdP. But ventricular tachycardia and TdP can cause sudden death without preceding warning symptoms. If there are predisposing underlying medical conditions, symptoms resulting from those may be seen.

> *TdP and sudden death can occur without any warning symptoms.*

Diagnosis

QTc is the best currently available EKG measurement to predict risk of TdP. The EKG may show premature ventricular contractions and short–long–short RR intervals immediately before an episode of TdP but these are not clinically useful for predicting future risk.

The QT is measured from the beginning of the QRS complex to the end of the T wave. Automatic EKG machines calculate the QT interval from the earliest Q wave in any lead to the last T wave in any lead. Since the QT interval is variable across leads, the automated QT interval is often longer than the QT interval measured in any given lead. The QT interval is inversely proportional to the heart rate and so has to be corrected to obtain the corrected QT interval (QTc). The most common formula is Bazett's, which is calculated by dividing the QT interval by the square root of the RR interval (QT/$\sqrt{RR}$). At the extremes of the heart rate range however, it results in error necessitating other formulae, such as Hodges formula (QTc = QT + 1.75 [HR−60]). A QT nomogram (QT versus heart rate) may be used to accurately predict risk of TdP [8].

The JT interval should be used instead of the QT interval in the case of a ventricular conduction defect so that the widened QRS does not affect the QTc length [9]. The point where QRS ends and the ST segment begins is the J point. If the end of the T wave is indistinct, the intersection of a tangent to the steepest slope of the T wave and the baseline should be used (see figure).

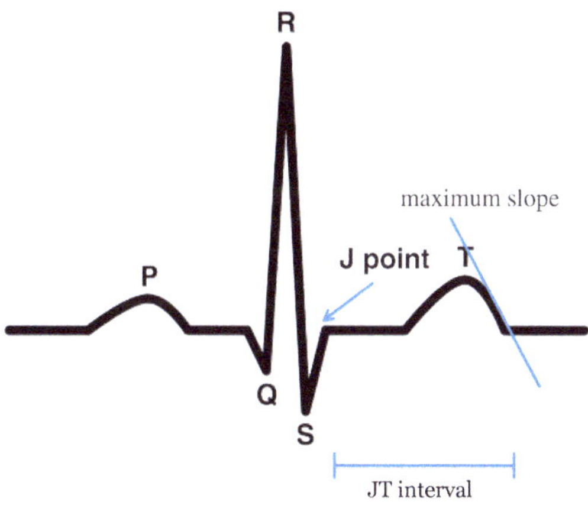

As a rough guide, the normal QT interval is approximately half the RR interval if the heart rate is approximately 60 beats/min. In clinical practice, the calculated QTc can be used especially if the QTc is normal since automated measurement is likely to overestimate and not underestimate the interval. If the QTc is significantly abnormal, then the automated measurement should be verified manually. Ideally the QT should be measured in multiple chest leads and averaged. But if only one lead is used, the QT should be estimated in the lead with the longest QT interval, usually V3, V2, or II. If heart rate is higher or lower than 60 beats/min and the QT interval is important for clinical risk prediction, then it should be corrected for heart rate using one of the earlier formulas.

If at all feasible, the EKG should be obtained during the time when the maximum serum level of the medication in question is expected.

Automated QT measurements can overestimate the interval; if abnormal, manually measure the QT in lead V3 and correct for heart rate.

Management

There are no clear guidelines for EKG monitoring on psychotropic medications. Routine EKG monitoring is usually not necessary for most psychotropic agents. Psychotropic agents are less likely than other drug classes such as antiarrhythmics to significantly prolong QTc. Prolongation usually occurs in the presence of other risk factors.

Some experts recommend performing an EKG before patients are started on higher risk medications like citalopram, ziprasidone, pimozide, or thioridazine though this is not a universal recommendation. It is advisable to perform an EKG before starting these medications in the presence of a second risk factor. If the QTc is already above normal (440 ms in males and 450 ms in females), alternate medications are preferred. During antiarrhythmic treatment initiation, measuring potassium and magnesium levels and maintaining at high normal levels is recommended. However, no such recommendation exists for psychotropic medications.

If baseline EKG was done and QTc was normal, an EKG should be repeated 4 weeks after initiation or when a steady medication dose is reached. It should also be repeated when dose is increased. There is no clear threshold over which the risk for torsades increases. But generally if the QTc >500 ms, most experts recommend stopping the drug. If the QTc change is >60 ms from baseline but is still <500 ms, stopping the drug should be considered.

Other risk factors for prolonged QTc, such as serum electrolyte imbalance, should be eliminated if QTc prolongation is seen during psychotropic treatment. Also, the patient should be made clearly aware of the risk of combining these agents with other medications such as antibiotics that can also prolong QTc.

Psychotropic agents generally cause significant QTc prolongation only in the presence of a second risk factor; key recommendation is to avoid higher risk medications in those with other risk factors.

In the absence of risk factors, it is not necessary to routinely measure EKG before and during psychotropic treatment but can be considered for ziprasidone and citalopram.

If EKG is obtained, repeat in 4 weeks and consider stopping the medication for >60 ms change from baseline or >500 ms QTc.

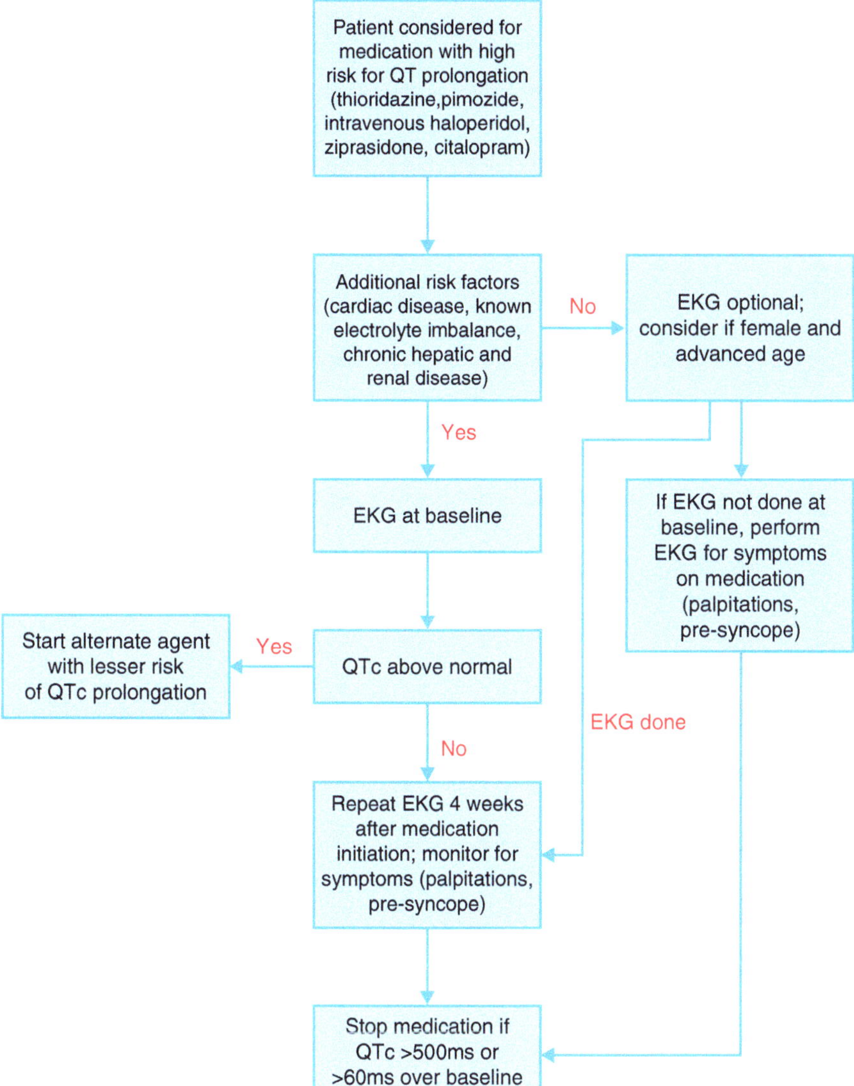

References

1. Beach SR, Celano CM, Noseworthy PA, Januzzi JL, Huffman JC. QTc prolongation, torsades de pointes, and psychotropic medications. Psychosomatics. 2013;54(1):1–13.
2. Glassman AH, Bigger Jr JT. Antipsychotic drugs: prolonged QTc interval, torsade de pointes, and sudden death. Am J Psychiatry. 2001;158(11):1774–82.
3. Strom BL, Eng SM, Faich G, Reynolds RF, D'Agostino RB, Ruskin J, et al. Comparative mortality associated with ziprasidone and olanzapine in real-world use among 18,154 patients with schizophrenia: The Ziprasidone Observational Study of Cardiac Outcomes (ZODIAC). Am J Psychiatry. 2011;168(2):193–201.

4. Leucht S, Cipriani A, Spineli L, Mavridis D, Örey D, Richter F, et al. Comparative efficacy and tolerability of 15 antipsychotic drugs in schizophrenia: a multiple-treatments meta-analysis. Lancet. 2013;382(9896):951–62.
5. Caccia S, Pasina L, Nobili A. New atypical antipsychotics for schizophrenia: iloperidone. Drug Des Devel Ther. 2010;4:33–48.
6. Janicak PG, Winans EA. Paliperidone ER: a review of the clinical trial data. Neuropsychiatr Dis Treat. 2007;3(6):869–97.
7. US Food and Drug Adminstration. FDA Drug Safety Communication: revised recommendations for Celexa (citalopram bromide) related to a potential risk of abnormal heart rhythms with high doses. http://www.fda.gov/drugs/drugsafety/ucm297391.htm. Accessed Oct 14, 2016.
8. Chan A, Isbister GK, Kirkpatrick CM, Dufful SB. Drug-induced QT prolongation and torsades de pointes: evaluation of a QT nomogram. QJM. 2007;100(10):609–15.
9. Zhou SH, Wong S, Rautaharju PM, Karnik N, Calhoun HP. Should the JT rather than the QT interval be used to detect prolongation of ventricular repolarization? An assessment in normal conduction and in ventricular conduction defects. J Electrocardiol. 1992;25(Suppl):131–6.

Chapter 9
Non-QT Conduction Abnormalities

Atrioventricular (AV) block is an interruption in the normal conduction of impulses from atria to the ventricles. Bundle branch block is a disruption in the conduction of impulses in one of the two bundles in the ventricles.

Pathology

First-degree AV block is slowed conduction without any missed beats. This is the type more likely to be seen as an adverse effect of psychotropic medications. In second-degree AV block, some atrial impulses do not reach the ventricle. Third-degree AV block is complete dissociation of atrial and ventricular impulses. First-degree block has good prognosis. Second-degree block can convert into a third-degree block, which has the potential to be fatal.

The prognosis of bundle branch block depends on the associated cardiac condition.

Etiology

AV block can be physiologic due to increased vagal tone as occurs with sleep and increased athletic activity. Most common pathologic causes for both AV block and bundle branch blocks are conditions that cause structural or ischemic heart disease. AV block can also be caused by medications (e.g., calcium channel blockers, beta blockers, antiarrhythmics).

© Springer International Publishing AG 2017

A. Annamalai, *Medical Management of Psychotropic Side Effects*,

DOI 10.1007/978-3-319-51026-2_9

Psychotropic Medications and Conduction Abnormalities

Tricyclic antidepressants (TCAs) are associated with both AV block and bundle branch block. The AV block is usually first but can be second degree. Any conduction delay is usually with drug overdose. It is rare at therapeutic doses but there is a small increase in risk in those with preexisting heart disease [1]. Since TCAs also prolong QTc and cause orthostatic hypotension, overall cardiovascular risk is increased. Conduction abnormalities are reversible on stopping the TCA.

Lithium has an effect on the sinus node and myocardium [2]. There are case reports of first-degree AV block even at therapeutic doses, though it is much more common with toxicity. Rare cases of complete heart block have been reported. The effect can occur at any stage of treatment. Arrhythmia from lithium appears to be reversible on cessation of medication or correction of toxicity.

The principal arrhythmic effect of antipsychotics is the QTc prolongation.

> ***Lithium and TCAs cause conduction delays mainly with toxicity but can rarely occur at therapeutic doses.***

Beta-blockers (e.g., propranolol) cause an expected decrease in resting heart rate. The small doses used for anxiety do not generally cause symptomatic bradycardia, especially in healthy people with no cardiac disease.

Clinical Features

Patients with first-degree AV block usually have no symptoms and the conduction abnormality is discovered only on EKG. Patients with second-degree AV block may have palpitations, fatigue, dizziness, and dyspnea. Patients with third-degree AV block almost certainly have some or many of these symptoms. Patients with bundle branch block will have symptoms related to the underlying condition, e.g., ischemia.

> ***First-degree AV block is asymptomatic and higher degree AV blocks may be associated with symptoms; symptoms of bundle branch blocks are due to the underlying condition.***

Diagnosis

First-degree AV block manifests as a PR interval >200 ms on the electrocardiogram (EKG). The PR interval measures both atrial depolarization and conduction through the ventricular system. Second-degree AV block manifests as a dropped ventricular beat (QRS) that is either preceded by progressive PR prolongation (type I) or occurs without any PR prolongation (type II). In third-degree AV block, the EKG shows complete dissociation of atrial (P) and ventricular (QRS) waves.

Bundle branch block has specific EKG criteria. In both right and left bundle branch block, the QRS is wide (>120 ms) and there are changes in V1 and V6 (see Chapter 11 for criteria). Often, there is incomplete block or other nonspecific conduction delays with some widening of QRS (100–110 ms). Nonspecific T wave flattening may also be seen on lithium treatment.

> ***Diagnosis of conduction abnormalities is primarily by EKG findings.***

Management

In patients with preexisting conduction abnormalities or other cardiac disease, it may be prudent to avoid TCAs and lithium as first-line treatment. In patients at higher risk, including prior ischemia with bundle branch block, it may be preferable to use a selective serotonin reuptake inhibitor (SSRI) unless there is a compelling indication for the TCA. Lithium may not be easily substituted and so can be used if clearly indicated. The risk of conduction abnormalities at therapeutic doses is small and any conduction abnormality with lithium is more likely to be a milder degree AV block.

For patients with preexisting cardiac disease, a baseline EKG is recommended before starting TCAs or lithium. For patients without cardiac disease, there is no clear consensus. Some experts recommend baseline as well as yearly EKG monitoring on TCAs especially if higher doses are used. For lithium, some experts recommend baseline EKG in older patients. For patients either on TCAs or lithium, EKG should be done for onset of new symptoms, occurrence of new cardiac disease, or suspected toxicity.

As mentioned earlier, the most likely abnormality to be seen with psychotropic medications is nonspecific conduction delays or mild AV block. If first-degree AV block is detected on medication, it can be continued if patient is asymptomatic. Periodic EKGs should be done. If higher degrees of AV block are found, medication should be stopped and patients should be referred for additional cardiology evaluation and treatment. In rare cases of third-degree AV block, a temporary pacemaker may be necessary until the abnormality reverses. If patients develop new bundle branch blocks, they should be referred to a cardiologist to rule out other etiologies.

There is no clear need for baseline EKG or periodic monitoring with TCA or lithium in patients without cardiac disease.

EKG monitoring in those with cardiac disease should be at least yearly and medication should be stopped for new conduction abnormalities.

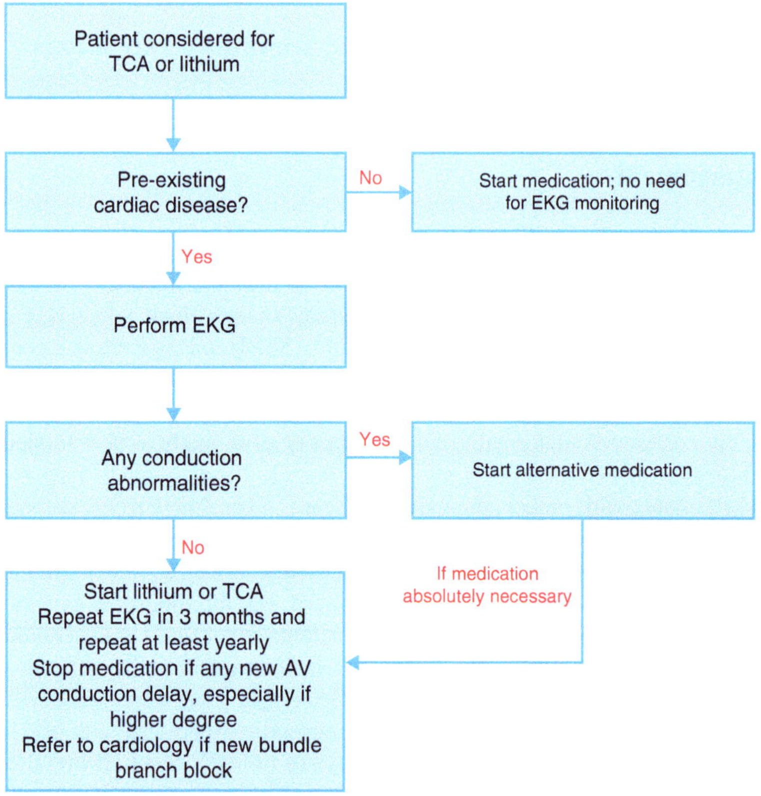

References

1. Roose SP, Glassman AH, Giardina EG, Walsh BT, Woodring S, Bigger JT. Tricyclic antidepressants in depressed patients with cardiac conduction disease. Arch Gen Psychiatry. 1987;44(3):273–5.
2. Oudit GY, Korley V, Backx PH, Dorian P. Lithium-induced sinus node disease at therapeutic concentrations: linking lithium-induced blockade of sodium channels to impaired pacemaker activity. Can J Cardiol. 2007;23(3):229–32.

Chapter 10
Peripheral Edema

Introduction

Edema is a clinical apparent increase in interstitial fluid. The interstitial fluid expansion can be generalized or localized. The prevalence depends on the specific etiology.

Pathology

Two basic processes in the occurrence of edema are extravasation of fluid from capillaries to the interstitium and retention of sodium and water by the kidneys. Edema usually is clinically apparent after 2–3 L of fluid accumulation in the interstitium. The severity of edema depends on the underlying etiology.

Etiology

See table for major causes of peripheral edema.

Major causes of edema

Serious medical conditions
Congestive heart failure
Cirrhosis of liver
Renal disease/nephrotic syndrome
Low albumin due to malnutrition or protein-losing enteropathy
Venous thrombosis, cellulitis (unilateral, localized and presents acutely)

(continued)

© Springer International Publishing AG 2017
A. Annamalai, *Medical Management of Psychotropic Side Effects*,
DOI 10.1007/978-3-319-51026-2_10

(continued)

Other medical conditions
Chronic venous insufficiency
Hypothyroidism
Postlymphatic dissection (unilateral, localized)
Nonpsychotropic medications (nonsteroidal anti-inflammatory agents, calcium channel blockers, vasodilators, thiazolidinediones, estrogen-containing agents
Physiologic
Pregnancy
Premenstrual syndrome
Idiopathic—seen in premenopausal females with no medical conditions

Psychotropic Medications and Edema

The most commonly accepted mechanism is capillary vasodilation from alpha-1 adrenergic blockade though water retention through activation of renin–aldosterone system is also postulated.

Among psychotropic agents, antipsychotics are most commonly associated with edema. The estimated prevalence is low at 1–3% [1]. The antipsychotics most commonly implicated are risperidone, olanzapine, and quetiapine [1]. Cases have been reported for chlorpromazine, haloperidol, paliperidone, clozapine also. The onset of edema is usually within 4 weeks of starting medication and occurs more commonly in females. In several patients, the medication had to be stopped due to severe or painful edema that interfered with functioning. All cases reported reversibility of edema with discontinuation of medication.

Among mood stabilizers, lithium has been reported to cause pedal edema by enhancing sodium retention [2] and in this case series, the edema spontaneously resolved in some cases though lithium was continued. Valproate has been associated with pedal edema both when used alone and in combination with antipsychotics. Among antidepressants, trazodone has been reported to cause dose-dependent reversible edema [3].

> *Prevalence of psychotropic medication-induced edema is low; antipsychotic agents are most commonly implicated.*

Psychotropic medications causing edema

Antipsychotics	
Risperidone, olanzapine, quetiapine (more likely)	
Chlorpromazine, haloperidol, clozapine, ziprasidone (less likely)	
Mood stabilizers	
Valproate, carbamazepine, lithium	
Antidepressants	
Trazodone	
Citalopram (in combination with an antipsychotic)	

Clinical Features

Edema is termed "pitting" when there is indentation following pressure in the area of increased swelling. Most etiologies cause pitting edema and the degree of pitting depends on severity of the edema. In milder cases of edema, only dependent regions of the body such as lower extremities may have clinically apparent edema. When edema is more widespread, patients may have shortness of breath or abdominal distension.

Edema from underlying medical conditions may be gradual (e.g., chronic heart failure, cirrhosis) or acute (e.g., venous thrombosis, which is often associated with pain and redness).

Medication-induced edema is acute in onset and correlates with initiation of medication. It ranges from mild-dependent swelling to a more generalized edema.

> ***Medication-induced edema usually occurs within 4 weeks of exposure; it can be mild or severe.***

Diagnosis

When there is no known underlying medical condition to explain the edema, further workup is necessary to rule out undiagnosed heart, liver, or kidney failure. A good history can screen for these conditions, whether acute or chronic. Laboratory tests appropriate for initial screening include liver function tests, basic metabolic profile, serum albumin, thyroid function tests. They may be referred for electrocardiogram or echocardiogram if there is suspicion for cardiac disease.

> ***Lab testing is done mainly to rule out other common and treatable etiologies.***

Management

Since edema can be from many etiologies and prevalence with psychotropic medications is low, underlying medical conditions should be ruled out. New onset concurrent symptoms such as shortness of breath or abdominal distension warrant a thorough medical evaluation. If the symptoms are acute in onset or unilateral, an urgent evaluation may be indicated. If onset is gradual and there are no alarm symptoms, screening for liver, kidney, and thyroid dysfunction can be done on an outpatient basis.

Medications, both psychotropic and nonpsychotropic agents should be reviewed. If the onset of edema corresponds to initiation of a psychotropic agent, management depends on whether the edema is mild or moderate-severe and interferes with physical functioning. Generally mild edema does not need any intervention and can be monitored. If edema is severe, medication should be stopped as a trial. If edema resolves off medication, a different agent that is less commonly associated with edema should be used instead. Diuretics can be used to reduce edema but it is generally preferable to stop the offending medication. If the edema does not resolve off the medication, other etiologies should be considered and patient should be referred to their primary care provider.

> *Underlying medical conditions should be ruled out before attributing edema to psychotropic medications.*
>
> *Mild psychotropic-induced edema does not need any intervention; if edema is severe, it is preferable to stop the offending medication.*

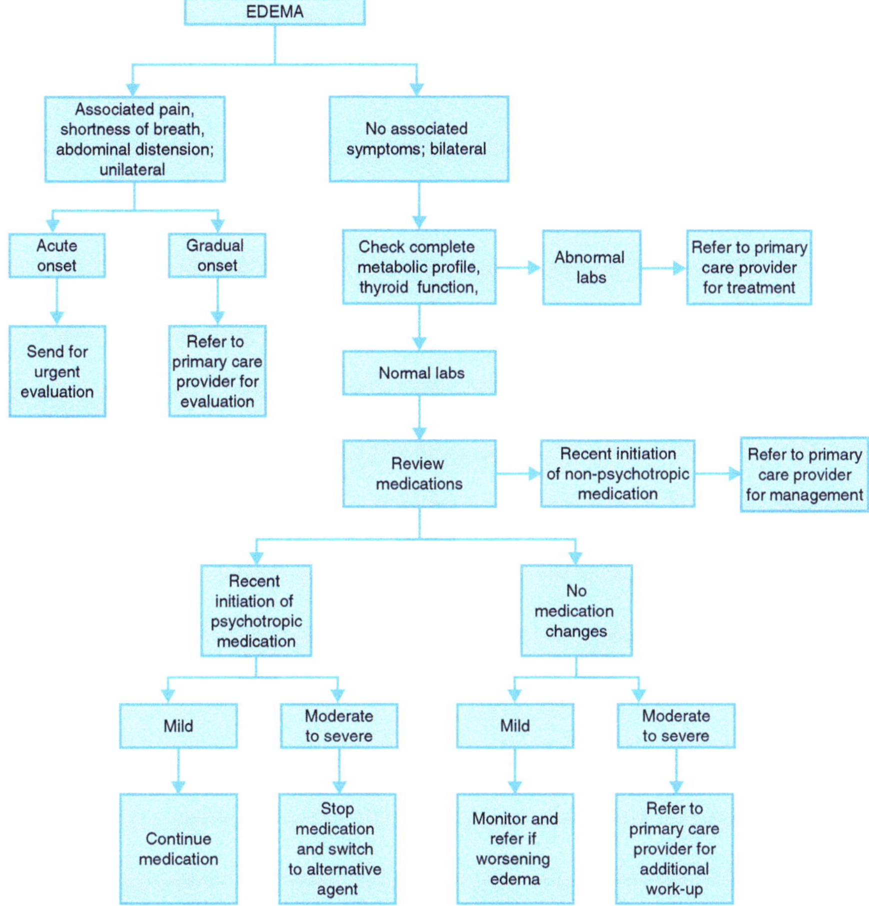

References

1. Chen HJ, Lin ST, Hsu HC, Cheng KD, Tsang HY. Paliperidone-related peripheral edema: a case report and review of the literature. J Clin Psychopharmacol. 2014;34(2):269–71.
2. Demers R, Heninger G. Pretibial edema and sodium retention during lithium carbonate treatment. JAMA. 1970;214(10):1845–8.
3. Barrnett J, Frances A, Kocsis J, Brown R, Mann JJ. Peripheral edema associated with trazodone: a report of ten cases. J Clin Psychopharmacol. 1985;5(3):161–4.

Chapter 11
Appendix: Miscellaneous Electrocardiographic Abnormalities

Many incidental EKG abnormalities may be seen when screening patients before medication initiation or monitoring patients on psychotropic medications. These EKG findings may sometimes need immediate attention or referral to a medical provider for additional workup. To perform this triage, it is important to understand some principles of EKG interpretation.

An EKG should always be interpreted in the context of current symptoms. If EKG is performed for routine screening, as is usually the case in a psychiatric outpatient setting, patient is asymptomatic. This is a key factor in determining whether the patient is experiencing an acute cardiac event. Whenever available, comparison should be made with old EKGs to determine if any change has occurred.

Automated measurements by EKG machines are reliable but have limitations. Also, final clinical interpretation requires other factors such as patient's clinical status and underlying medical conditions.

Some tips are listed in the following tables to differentiate normal and abnormal EKG tracings:

Comparison of normal and abnormal tracing of individual EKG components

	Normal pattern	Conditions associated with abnormalities
P wave (right followed by left atrial depolarization) (<0.12 s or 3 small boxes wide and <0.25 mV or 2.5 small boxes high)	Notched in limb leads and biphasic in V1	Widened P wave in right atrial enlargement Tall peaked P wave in left atrial enlargement
PR interval—from beginning of P to beginning of QRS(atrial depolarization and A–V conduction) (0.12 s or 3 small boxes to 0.2 s or 5 small boxes)	Shorter at high heart rates without other abnormalities	Short PR—WPW syndrome Prolonged PR—AV conduction delay

(continued)

© Springer International Publishing AG 2017

A. Annamalai, *Medical Management of Psychotropic Side Effects*,
DOI 10.1007/978-3-319-51026-2_11

(continued)

	Normal pattern	Conditions associated with abnormalities
QRS—initial negative deflection is Q; first positive deflection is R; negative deflection after R is S (ventricular depolarization) (0.06 s or 1.5 small boxes to 0.1 s or 2.5 small boxes)	R wave progresses in amplitude from V1 to V6	Widened QRS in bundle branch block Poor R wave progression in conditions that disrupt left ventricular conduction
ST segment—from end of QRS to beginning of T (between ventricular depolarization and repolarization)	Normally slightly concave; can be rapidly upsloping in tachycardia	Convex elevation in pericarditis, myocarditis, infarction, LBBB Depression in ischemia
T wave (ventricular depolarization)	Slow upstroke and rapid downstroke; generally smooth; usually concordant with QRS	Symmetric inversion in ischemia/infarction Tall with conduction abnormalities
QT interval—beginning of QRS to end of T (ventricular depolarization and repolarization) (<0.44 s in males and <0.45 s in females)	Shorter at faster heart rates and so corrected QT is calculated	Prolonged in electrolyte imbalance, structural anomalies, medication induced Can be falsely prolonged with conduction delay and QRS widening

Differentiating ischemic and nonischemic ST-T patterns

	Nonischemic	Ischemia/infarction
T wave inversion	More likely in right precordial leads (V1-V3), asymmetry maintained Causes: Juvenile variant, athletes, ventricular hypertrophy, bundle branch block	More likely in left precordial leads (V4–V6), becomes symmetric (>0.1 mV in 2 anatomically contiguous leads) Causes: Postischemic state
ST elevation	More likely to be concave Causes: Early repolarization, left ventricular hypertrophy, hyperkalemia, pericarditis, myocarditis	More likely to be convex (>1 mm above baseline at J point) Causes: Myocardial ischemia or infarction, LBBB
ST depression	More likely to be upsloping Causes: Ventricular hypertrophy	More likely to be downsloping or horizontal (>0.5 mm below baseline measured 0.08 s after J point) Causes: Myocardial ischemia
Q wave	More likely to be isolated Causes: Normal variant in V1, V2, III, aVL, aVF, Ventricular hypertrophy, LBBB	Often accompanied by T inversion In 2 contiguous leads (≥30 ms, ≥1 mm deep and usually ≥1/3rd QRS amplitude) Causes: Postmyocardial infarction
Tall T wave (>10 mm precordial leads and >5 mm limb leads)	Other findings associated with cause Causes: Early repolarization, hyperkalemia, LVH, LBBB	Other findings of infarction Causes: Acute phase of myocardial infarction

EKG findings in selected cardiac conditions

Physiologic or pathologic condition	EKG abnormality
Right bundle branch block (RBBB)	RSR' in V1,V2 + wide QRS (>120 ms) and deep S in V6
Left bundle branch block (LBBB)	RR' in V5,V6 + wide QRS (>120 ms) and QS in V1,V2
Incomplete bundle branch block	QRS wide but <120 ms with BBB pattern
Left anterior fascicular block (LAFB)	Left axis deviation (LAD) + positive QRS in I, negative QRS in aVF + QRS <120 ms
Left posterior fascicular block (LPFB)	Right axis deviation (RAD) + negative QRS in I, positive QRS in aVF + QRS <120 ms
Intraventricular conduction delay	QRS>110 ms without typical BBB pattern
First-degree AV block	PR>200 ms
Second-degree AV block	Dropped QRS after progressive PR lengthening (type I) OR dropped QRS after consistent PR intervals (type II)
Third-degree AV block	P & QRS disparate
Left ventricular hypertrophy (LVH)	S in V1 + R in V5 or V6 $\geq$35 mm
Right ventricular hypertrophy (RVH)	R in V1 + S in V5 or V6 >10 mm
Sinus arrhythmia	Variation in P–P interval >120 ms
Atrial fibrillation	No discrete P + variable RR intervals
<u>Past ischemia</u> ST elevation myocardial infarction (STEMI) Non-ST myocardial infarction (NSTEMI)	Reduced R amplitude + new or deeper Q + T inversion ST depression + T inversion

Section IV
Endocrine System

Chapter 12
Hyperprolactinemia

Hyperprolactinemia is a state of elevated levels of serum prolactin (PRL). The prevalence in the general population is not well known. Prolactin-secreting tumors have an annual incidence of 3/100,000 population. Normal PRL levels are about 15–30 µg/L in adults.

Pathology

Prolactin is synthesized and secreted from the lactotroph cells in the anterior pituitary gland. PRL secretion is pulsatile and serum levels vary depending on time of day. Peak serum levels are usually in the early morning hours of sleep. Secretion is regulated by an inhibitory mechanism via a dopamine-mediated suppression. Dopamine type 2 (D2) receptors in the pituitary mediate PRL inhibition. The hypothalamic thyrotropin releasing hormone (TRH) increases secretion of PRL.

An important physiologic role of prolactin is to induce and maintain lactation. It also suppresses reproduction so that physiologic maternal lactation is not interrupted. PRL levels rise during pregnancy and then decrease at the end of pregnancy and after delivery with intermittent elevations during breastfeeding. PRL inhibits reproductive function at multiple levels from the hypothalamus to the ovaries and testicles. Changes caused by PRL reduce libido and fertility in both men and women.

PRL also has other metabolic effects that are geared to sustain lactation. It acts on centers in the brain involved in parenting behaviors and appetite stimulation. It also stimulates gastrointestinal absorption of calcium and mobilization of calcium from bone.

The main effect of a sustained elevation in PRL is reduction of fertility in both men and women. Elevated PRL for many years may affect calcium homeostasis and bone health.

© Springer International Publishing AG 2017   85
A. Annamalai, *Medical Management of Psychotropic Side Effects*,
DOI 10.1007/978-3-319-51026-2_12

Etiology

See table for causes of hyperprolactinemia. The major physiologic causes of PRL elevation are pregnancy and lactation. Both physical and psychological stress can also increase PRL levels. Chronic renal and liver failure can result in decreased peripheral clearance of PRL.

Prolactinomas are prolactin-secreting adenomas in the pituitary. They are classified as microadenomas if the size is <1 cm or macroadenomas if size is >1 cm. Less commonly, other pituitary tumors and hypothalamic lesions cause some PRL elevation.

Many antipsychotics and antidepressants cause hyperprolactinemia. Other medications that cause PRL elevation also act by inhibiting dopamine synthesis or release. Oral contraceptives may cause a slight elevation in PRL levels.

Causes of hyperprolactinemia

Physiologic	Pregnancy
	Lactation
	Nipple stimulation
	Sexual intercourse
	Stress
Hypothalamic disorders	Tumors
	Infiltrative disorders
	Head trauma
Pituitary disorders	Prolactin-secreting tumors
	Tumors compressing the pituitary stalk
Other endocrine disorders	Hypothyroidism
	Acromegaly
Systemic illnesses	Chronic renal failure
	Liver cirrhosis
	Seizure disorder
Chest wall lesions	Chest wall trauma
	Herpes Zoster
Drugs	Antipsychotics
	Antidepressants
	Antihypertensives (methyldopa, reserpine, verapamil)
	Opiates
	Gastrointestinal (cimetidine, metoclopramide)
	Hormones (estrogens, antiandrogens)

Psychotropic Medications and Hyperprolactinemia

Any medication with activity against dopamine receptors can cause PRL elevation by inhibiting the normal dopamine-mediated suppression of PRL. The estimated incidence of dopamine antagonist-treated hyperprolactinemia for women is

8.7/100,000 person-years and for men 1.4/100,000 person-years [1]. For patients who use high-potency dopamine-2 receptor blocking agents, incidence as high as 70% has been reported [2].

Antipsychotics increase prolactin by antagonizing D2 receptors in tuberoinfundibular pathway in the brain.

Among antipsychotics, the typical agents are more likely to raise PRL than the atypical agents. Risperidone is an exception and causes even higher PRL elevation than typical antipsychotics. One mechanism is thought to be higher receptor occupancy at the level of the pituitary gland. See table for differential risk with different antipsychotics. Aripiprazole may even lower PRL due to its partial dopamine agonist and antagonist properties. Almost all antidepressants can raise PRL via serotonergic pathways but the increase is small and clinical symptoms are rare [3]. The PRL elevation from antidepressants only assumes clinical relevance if they are administered with prolactin-inducing antipsychotics.

Antipsychotic induced prolactin elevation

Risperidone, paliperidone	+++
High-potency typical antipsychotics (e.g., haloperidol, fluphenazine)	++
Clozapine, olanzapine, quetiapine, ziprasidone, lurasidone, asenapine, iloperidone, low-potency typical antipsychotics (e.g., chlorpromazine)	+/−
Aripiprazole	− −

The degree of PRL elevation may indicate whether the etiology is a prolactin-secreting tumor or a secondary cause. Secondary causes of PRL elevation generally cause PRL elevation <100 µg/L though higher levels can be seen with risperidone and some high-potency typical antipsychotics. Levels up to 300 µg/mL have been noted especially with risperidone. Prolactinomas usually cause PRL levels >100 µg/mL though microadenomas may only raise PRL levels to <100 µg/L. Nonlactotrope pituitary masses and hypothalamic lesions usually raise PRL levels to <100 µg/mL.

Prolactin <100 µg/mL is unlikely to be due to a prolactinoma.

Some antipsychotics can raise prolactin >100 µg/mL.

Females are more likely to both develop higher PRL elevation from medications and to experience clinical symptoms. PRL elevation usually is seen soon after treatment initiation but clinical effects may take several weeks to develop. The PRL elevation is dose dependent though large increases can be seen even at relatively low doses. Stopping the medication brings the level back to normal within 2–3 weeks.

> ***Antipsychotic-induced hyperprolactinemia is potency and dose dependent. Stopping medication quickly reverses the prolactinemia.***

Clinical Features

Hyperprolactinemia from any cause is unlikely before menarche but if it occurs, it can lead to primary amenorrhea. After menarche, it leads to oligomenorrhea and ultimately to secondary amenorrhea. Galactorrhea and infertility are other hallmarks of hyperprolactinemia in women. The galactorrhea is usually bilateral and spontaneous but may be unilateral and expressible only with manual stimulation. In postmenopausal women, symptoms such as vaginal dryness, dyspareunia, and loss of libido may be exacerbated. In men, diminished libido is the usual presenting symptom. The gonadotropin suppression also leads to reduced testosterone, impotence, and oligospermia causing male infertility. Galactorrhea occurs much less commonly in men than in women. In both sexes, there is reasonable evidence that sustained elevations in PRL lead to loss of bone mineral density and osteopenia over the long term. If there is a large prolactinoma, patients may present with symptoms related to optic nerve compression such as diplopia or vision loss.

> ***<u>Common symptoms of hyperprolactinemia.</u>***
>
> ***Women: Amenorrhea, breast engorgement and/or galactorrhea, infertility.***
>
> ***Men: Loss of libido, erectile dysfunction.***

Diagnosis

In patients with hyperprolactinemia, the history and physical exam serve to differentiate between a PRL-secreting pituitary tumor and secondary cause of elevated PRL. Physiologic causes such as pregnancy should be ruled out. Laboratory tests should include thyroid function tests to rule out hypothyroidism and liver and kidney function tests to rule out decreased clearance of PRL.

PRL is ideally measured as a fasting morning level. Since the PRL secretion is pulsatile and varies widely in some individuals, it may be necessary to measure levels on more than one occasion. An unexpected falsely high or falsely low level should be repeated. Basal levels are generally <20 µg/L.

If secondary causes including drugs are unlikely, then pituitary magnetic resonance imaging (MRI) is done to rule out a prolactinoma. PRL level reduction in response to dopamine agonists cannot be used as a diagnostic tool for prolactinomas as elevated PRL from other causes also responds to medical therapy.

> ***History is important in differentiating primary and secondary causes.***
>
> ***Pregnancy test in females and thyroid, liver, and kidney function tests in both males and females should be done before further workup.***

Management

There is no need to routinely screen for prolactin in patients on antipsychotics. If patients report symptoms including infertility, PRL can be checked. If possible, the timing of PRL measurement should be consistent before and after medication to reliably assess for changes. Other treatable conditions should be eliminated by appropriate testing.

If elevated, dose reduction may help reduce PRL levels. If dose reduction is not tolerated or sufficient to reduce PRL levels, low-dose aripiprazole can be used adjunctively to decrease PRL levels. The effect seems to plateau after about 6 mg of aripiprazole and so there is no benefit in higher doses [4].

If patient does not desire fertility and is otherwise asymptomatic, medication can be continued in spite of elevated PRL. However, given the potential for bone loss over the long term, significantly high PRL levels may be an indication to switch to a different antipsychotic. There is no particular cutoff when the risk of osteopenia is significant but likely increases with PRL>100 µg/L and definitely with PRL>200 µg/L.

If the offending antipsychotic is deemed necessary, dopamine agonists such as bromocriptine and cabergoline can be considered to reduce PRL levels. If fertility is not desired, gonadal hormone replacement such as estrogen and testosterone will prevent bone loss though PRL level will remain high. These treatments should be started only in conjunction with an endocrinologist and when it is imperative to continue the antipsychotic.

If decision is made to stop the offending antipsychotic, PRL level should be checked 4–6 weeks later. If it remains high, patient should be referred for further evaluation to rule out coexisting prolactinoma. Treatment options for an identified prolactinoma include dopamine agonists and surgical removal.

Routine screening of prolactin in asymptomatic psychiatric patients is not necessary.

Dose reduction or adjunctive aripiprazole can be used to reduce prolactin in symptomatic patients and those who desire fertility.

In asymptomatic patients, intervention may be needed if prolactin >200 µg/L to prevent bone loss.

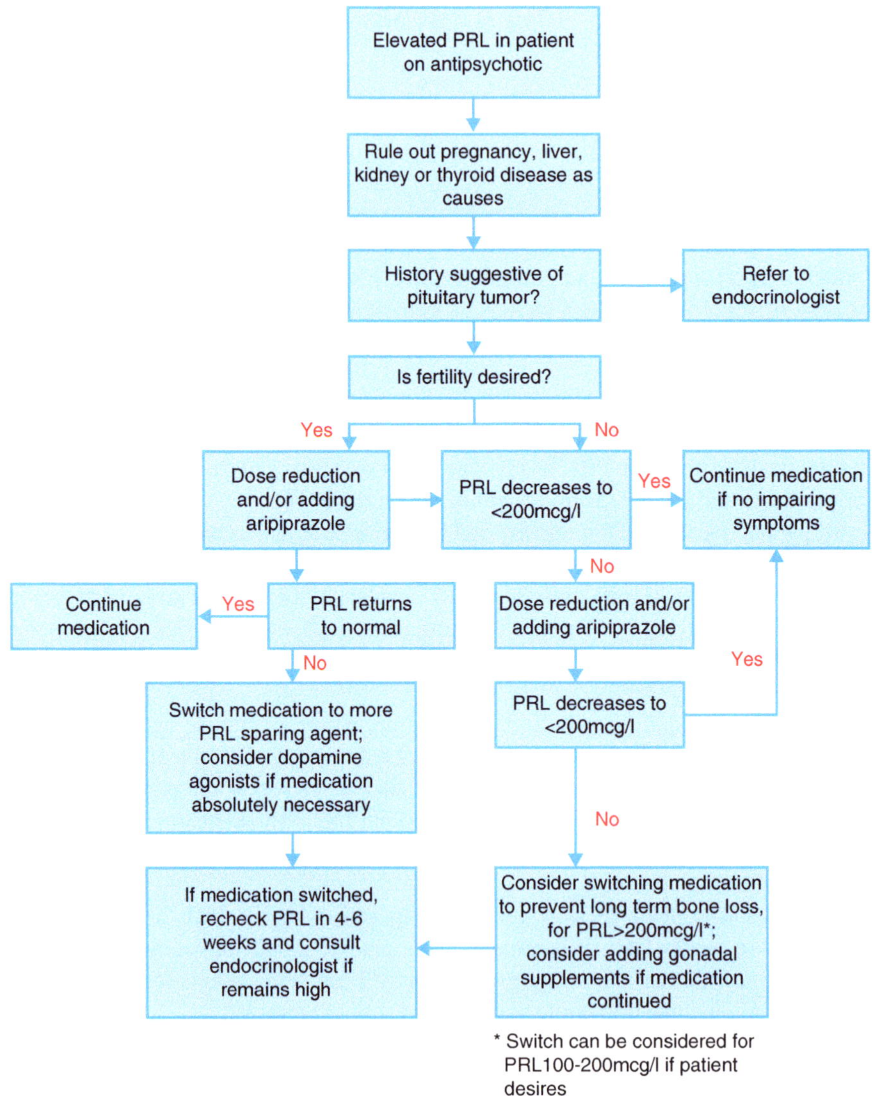

References

1. Kars M, Souverein PC, Herings RM, Romijn JA, Vandenbroucke JP, de Boer A, et al. Estimated age- and sex-specific incidence and prevalence of dopamine agonist-treated hyperprolactinemia. J Clin Endocrinol Metab. 2009;94(8):2729–34.
2. Montgomery J, Winterbottom E, Jessani M, Kohegyi E, Fulmer J, Seamonds B, et al. Prevalence of hyperprolactinemia in schizophrenia: association with typical and atypical antipsychotic treatment. J Clin Psychiatry. 2004;65(11):1491–8.
3. Coker F, Taylor D. Antidepressant-induced hyperprolactinaemia: incidence, mechanisms and management. CNS Drugs. 2010;24(7):563–74.
4. Yasui-Furukori N, Furukori H, Sugawara N, Fujii A, Kaneko S. Dose-dependent effects of adjunctive treatment with aripiprazole on hyperprolactinemia induced by risperidone in female patients with schizophrenia. J Clin Psychopharmacol. 2010;30(5):596–9.

Chapter 13
Thyroid Disorders

Hypothyroidism is a state of lowered thyroid hormone activity. Hyperthyroidism is a state of excessive thyroid function. The diagnosis is made primarily by laboratory testing since clinical manifestations are nonspecific. The diagnosis is made based on serum levels of thyroid hormones and thyroid stimulating hormone.

Pathology

The thyroid gland produces two hormones, thyroxine (T4) and triiodothyronine (T3). These hormones are critical for cell differentiation during development and to maintain homeostasis in adults. TSH, secreted by the anterior pituitary gland plays an important role in controlling the thyroid axis and is the most useful physiologic marker for thyroid function. The thyroid axis is an endocrine feedback loop. Thyrotropin releasing hormone (TRH) from the hypothalamus stimulates TSH release and TSH stimulates T4 and T3 release. TRH is the major regulator of TSH synthesis and secretion. When thyroid hormone levels are low, TRH-mediated secretion of TSH is enhanced and TSH levels rise. When thyroid hormone levels are high, TRH-mediated TSH secretion is reduced and TSH levels drop.

Iodine is necessary for thyroid hormone synthesis. Both thyroid hormones are produced by the thyroid gland but T4 is secreted at a much higher proportion than T3. Once released, most of the circulating hormones are bound to plasma proteins. Only the free hormones are biologically active in tissues. T4 is converted to the more potent T3 in the periphery. Circulating levels of free T3 are higher than free T4 though total T3 is less than total T4.

© Springer International Publishing AG 2017
A. Annamalai, *Medical Management of Psychotropic Side Effects*,
DOI 10.1007/978-3-319-51026-2_13

Etiology

In the United States, autoimmune disease is the most common cause of hypothyroidism with Hashimotos disease being the common variant. Iodine deficiency is a common cause of hypothyroidism in iodine-deficient regions of the world. Secondary causes are due to TRH or TSH deficiencies.

See table for causes of hypothyroidism.

Causes of hypothyroidism

Primary	Autoimmune (Hashimotos)
	Iatrogenic (surgical removal or radiation)
	Medications (lithium, contrast media, amiodarone, interferon)
	Iodine deficiency
	Infiltrative disorders
Secondary	Disorders causing hypopituitarism
	Hypothalamic disease
	Isolated TSH deficiency
Transient	Silent thyroiditis (postpartum)
	Post I^{131} treatment or subtotal thyroidectomy

The common causes of primary hyperthyroidism are Graves disease, toxic multinodular goiter, and toxic adenomas. Secondary causes of hyperthyroidism are TSH-secreting pituitary adenomas and thyroid hormone resistance syndrome. Subacute thyroiditis, silent thyroiditis, and drug-induced thyroiditis cause transient elevation of thyroid hormones due to follicular destruction. Some medications such as propranolol or salicylate displace thyroid hormone from serum binding protein and increase the free circulating hormone level; the thyroid axis transiently is perturbed but soon resets to the new steady state.

Psychotropic Medications and Thyroid Disorders

Lithium can affect thyroid function in a multitude of ways. It is concentrated in the thyroid gland and has the potential to disrupt both thyroid hormone formation and secretion. Lithium can also accelerate thyroid antibody formation. It does not cause but worsens thyroid autoimmunity. Studies have estimated clinical hypothyroidism in 8–19% patients versus 0.5–1.8% in the general population and subclinical hypothyroidism in 23% versus 10.4% in the general population [1]. In a large meta-analysis, the rate of hypothyroidism was about sixfold for those on lithium [2].

Lithium-induced hypothyroidism develops usually in weeks to months but can take years. Risk factors are female gender, older age, family history of thyroid disease. Most patients are asymptomatic and it is unclear if and when treatment should be initiated for hypothyroidism. There is no evidence that stopping lithium reverses the thyroid dysfunction but small studies have shown some normalization of TFTs upon lithium cessation [2]. It may be that in cases where lithium enhances thyroid autoimmunity, the thyroid dysfunction is irreversible.

There is at least a sixfold increased risk of hypothyroidism from lithium.

Stopping lithium often does not reverse the thyroid dysfunction.

Goiter, a diffuse enlargement of the thyroid gland, is reported in up to 40% patients on lithium [1]. The thyroid enlargement is in part due to the increase in TSH caused by thyroid hormone inhibition. Goiters are slow growing and may take years to develop. They can be asymptomatic or present with hypothyroidism or even hyperthyroidism. Lithium causes homogenous thyroid gland enlargement and these goiters are more like to cause hypo rather than hyperthyroidism. In late stages, goiters can become fibrotic at which point surgery may be the only treatment option. It is rare for lithium to be a cause of a clinically significant goiter.

Lithium rarely causes clinically significant goiter formation.

Even though lithium generally has a suppressive effect on the thyroid, there are case reports of hyperthyroidism also. Compared to hypothyroidism, it is more likely to occur earlier in the treatment course. The mechanism is unclear. It is either due to direct damage of thyroid cells causing thyroiditis or lithium-induced autoimmune-mediated hyperthyroidism [1]. In the case of thyroiditis, it may convert later to hypothyroidism. If lithium is stopped, it may reverse especially if thyroiditis is the pathology.

There are rare case reports of lithium-induced hyperthyroidism.

Other psychotropics may also interfere with thyroid function [3]. Antipsychotic medications, especially phenothiazines, induce autoantibody formation and may cause a hypothyroid state. Antidepressants (TCAs, SSRIs) and mood stabilizers (carbamazepine, valproate) also interfere with thyroid function but have little clinical impact.

Other psychotropic medications can interfere with thyroid function but rarely cause clinically significant hypothyroidism.

Clinical Features

The onset of symptoms is insidious and patients often do not become aware of symptoms until later stages. Common features of hypothyroidism are constipation, weight gain, menstrual abnormalities, and reduced libido. Skin changes and nonpitting edema are seen in later stages of the disease. Reduced cardiac function can lead to bradycardia. Rarely, neurologic symptoms occur. If a goiter is present, patients may complain of neck swelling.

See table for a complete list of symptoms.

Symptoms and signs of hypothyroidism

Symptoms	Signs
Fatigue	Coarse thickened skin Cool extremities Puffy face and hands Nonpitting peripheral edema
Dry skin, skin thickening, hair loss, brittle nails	Alopecia
Cold intolerance	Bradycardia
Constipation	Delayed deep tendon reflexes
Weight gain	Carpal tunnel syndrome
Poor memory and concentration	Pleural cavity effusions
Menorrhagia (or oligomenorrhea/amenorrhea)	Dementia, psychosis, reversible ataxia, encephalopathy
Dyspnea	
Paresthesias	
Voice and hearing changes	
Joint pains	

People with hyperthyroidism may show symptoms associated with psychiatric illness such as hyperactivity, mood dysregulation, anxiety, irritability, weakness and fatigue, insomnia, impaired concentration. Other symptoms are weight loss in spite of increased appetite, heat intolerance, palpitations, diarrhea, oligomenorrhea. Signs of hyperthyroidism include tachycardia, tremor, warm and moist skin, myopathy. If the hyperthyroidism is due to autoimmune Graves disease, lid lag or lid retraction is seen.

In patients with lithium-induced hypo or hyperthyroidism, symptoms may be difficult to distinguish from those of preexisting mood disorder.

Symptoms of hypothyroidism or hyperthyroidism, lithium induced or otherwise, may be difficult to distinguish from those of underlying depression and anxiety symptoms.

Diagnosis

Thyroid functions tests (TFTs) should be routinely checked during treatment with lithium. They should also be checked in the presence of any clinical symptoms. Hyperlipidemia, hyperprolactinemia, hyponatremia, and elevated creatine phosphokinase enzyme should also prompt screening for hypothyroidism. TFTs should also always be tested in patients with depression or anxiety especially in the presence of risk factors (other autoimmune disease or family history of thyroid disorders).

TSH should be the first step in screening for hypothyroidism. But testing should preferably be avoided during acute illness, as TSH can be falsely abnormal. If TSH is high, then hypothyroidism is suspected and free T4 (FT4) levels are measured. FT4 is preferable to total T4 as the former is not affected by changes in serum proteins. FT4 should not be used as the screening test as it can be normal in mild and subclinical thyroid disease. In a minority of cases of hyperthyroidism, T3 is high with a normal T4. Hence, if TSH is low and free T4 is normal, T3 should be measured. Free T3 levels can be measured but are not necessary for the diagnosis of hypothyroidism.

Once a diagnosis of hypo or hyperthyroidism is made, measuring autoantibodies—antithyroid peroxidase antibody (TPO), antithyroglobulin antibodies (Tg), and thyroid-stimulating immunoglobulin (TSI)—can be done to evaluate for autoimmune disease. Antithyroid antibodies are present in nearly all cases of autoimmune hypothyroidism; however, presence of antibodies does not rule out lithium-induced disease as lithium accelerates thyroid autoimmunity in those with preexisting antibodies.

TSH is the initial screening test; FT4 can be checked with TSH but not alone as a screening test.

Presence of thyroid autoantibodies does not reliably rule out lithium-induced thyroid disease and so antibody testing is optional.

Hypo or hyperthyroidism is divided into the following categories based on TSH and FT4 (and not based on clinical symptoms):

Clinical hypo or hyperthyroidism: Lab evidence of high TSH and low FT4 in hypothyroidism and low TSH and high FT4, FT3 in hyperthyroidism. TSH is usually >10 and <0.1 mU/L in hypo and hyperthyroidism, respectively.

Subclinical hypo or hyperthyroidism: In hypothyroidism, TSH is high (usually 4–10 mU/L) and FT4 is normal. A substantial portion of these patients develop overt hypothyroidism. The risk is higher with higher TSH values and if antithyroid antibodies are present. In hyperthyroidism, TSH is low (usually 0.1–0.5 mU/L) and both FT4 and FT3 are normal.

In sick euthyroid syndrome, TFT abnormalities are seen as a result of acute illness. In secondary hypothyroidism, both TSH and FT4 are low and in secondary hyperthyroidism, both TSH and FT4 are high.

Some conditions where the thyroid gland is inflamed such as postpartum thyroiditis can cause an initial hyperthyroid phase and then a temporary hypothyroid phase.

Categories of hypo and hyperthyroidism

Clinical	
Hypothyroidism	TSH high; FT4 low
Hyperthyroidism	TSH low; FT4, FT3 high
Subclinical	
Hypothyroidism	TSH high; FT4 normal
Hyperthyroidism	TSH low; FT4 normal
Secondary	
Hypothyroidism	TSH low; FT4 low
Hyperthyroidism	TSH high; FT4 high
Sick euthyroid syndrome	TSH usually high but may be low; FT4 low or high

> ***Categorization into clinical and subclinical hypothyroidism depends on FT4 level and not on presence or absence of clinical symptoms.***
>
> ***TFTs are not reliable markers of thyroid function during an acute nonthyroidal illness.***

A physical exam may reveal a goiter, which will be palpable as a homogenously enlarged thyroid gland. However, an exam is unreliable in accurately differentiating between homogenous enlargement and nodularity. Hence, any enlargement will require further testing such as ultrasound and fine needle aspiration cytology.

Management

In patients on lithium, TFTs are checked at the initiation of therapy. Some experts advocate checking for antithyroid antibodies at baseline to determine those at risk for developing autoimmune thyroid disease on lithium. During lithium therapy, TFTs should be checked 3 months after initiation and at least yearly thereafter. TSH is sufficient as a screening test. If abnormal, then FT4 should be checked. With mild TFT abnormalities, labs should be repeated in 6–8 weeks to rule out transient causes.

Hypothyroidism

For those patients with clinical hypothyroidism on lithium, the patient and clinician should decide if lithium should be continued. As noted earlier, the thyroid dysfunction may not be reversible even with stopping the lithium. Even if TFTs revert to normal, it may take several weeks and testing should not be done for at least 8 weeks after stopping lithium.

If lithium is continued, levothyroxine should be initiated. The duration of levothyroxine treatment is for the duration of the lithium treatment. The lithium dose does not need to be changed. Treatment is with thyroid hormone replacement. T4 is preferable to T3 as it has a longer half-life and is easier to administer. T3 replacement does not produce a consistent level of thyroid hormone in the serum. The starting T4 dosage is usually 25 µg/day. If dose increases are needed, dose adjustments are in increments of 12–25 µg/day. Monitoring treatment is by measurement of TSH, which should be measured 6 weeks after initiation of therapy and then every 3 months until steady TSH values are reached. Once the dose is stabilized, TSH can be measured every 6 months to a year. If there is a change in symptoms soon after T4 dose adjustment, T4 is also measured.

If patient is already on T3 for adjunctive treatment of depression, treatment with both T4 and T3 could be considered. There is no evidence that the combination treatment has advantages over T4 replacement [4] in patients with hypothyroidism, but in patients who also need treatment for depression, combination may be effective [5]. T4 alone as treatment for depression is not well documented.

For those patients with subclinical hypothyroidism on lithium, antibodies may be helpful to predict risk of conversion to overt hypothyroidism. Threshold for treatment is controversial. The benefits of treatment have to be weighed against the risks of excess thyroid replacement. Most experts recommend treatment if TSH >10 mU/L or if there are symptoms suggestive of hypothyroidism. Another recommended approach is to treat those patients who also have antithyroid antibodies as they are at higher risk for conversion to overt hypothyroidism. For patients with TSH in the 5–10 mU/L range, treatment can be deferred in the absence of symptoms or serum antibodies. However, if patients have residual mood symptoms, it is reasonable to initiate T4 replacement earlier in the course.

Hyperthyroidism

Hyperthyroidism from lithium is rare and so there are no clear guidelines for management. If thyroid antibodies are elevated indicating Graves disease, lithium still cannot be ruled out as a cause since it can induce autoimmunity in susceptible individuals.

For patients with subclinical hyperthyroidism, treatment is recommended if TSH <0.1 mU/L. If TSH is >0.1 mU/L <0.5 mU/L treatment is recommended for those at high risk for cardiac and skeletal complications as long-term thyroid excess increases risk for cardiac arrhythmias and bone loss.

Hyperthyroidism on lithium may reverse on stopping lithium if it is due to a destructive thyroiditis but may not if it is due to autoimmune disease. If lithium is continued, antithyroid drugs, radioiodine or in some cases, thyroidectomy may be needed. Long-acting beta blockers, such as propranolol, are useful in suppressing the adrenergic effects of excess thyroid hormone. It is best to refer patients to an endocrinologist for complete evaluation and treatment of hyperthyroidism.

Goiter

If a goiter is suspected, treatment recommendations depend on whether the patient is euthyroid, hypothyroid, or hyperthyroid. In hypothyroid patients, T4 replacement treats the biochemical deficiency and also prevents further enlargement of the goiter. There is no consensus on treatment of goiter for euthyroid patients though replacement is recommended in patients with significant enlargement. Since goiter is more likely due to other causes such as iodine deficiency or thyroiditis, these patients should be referred for further evaluation. Also, as thyroid enlargement may be due to other causes such as nodular disease or malignancy, a thorough evaluation is warranted.

TFTs should be checked routinely during lithium treatment.

Autoantibody testing is optional but may help determine risk of conversion to clinical thyroid disease in the presence of subclinical disease.

If lithium is stopped due to thyroid dysfunction, TFTs should be retested approximately 8 weeks later.

If lithium is continued, hypothyroidism should be treated with T4; patients should be referred for treatment of hyperthyroidism.

There is a lower threshold for treating subclinical thyroid disease in patients with preexisting persistent depression or anxiety.

A suspicion for goiter warrants a referral.

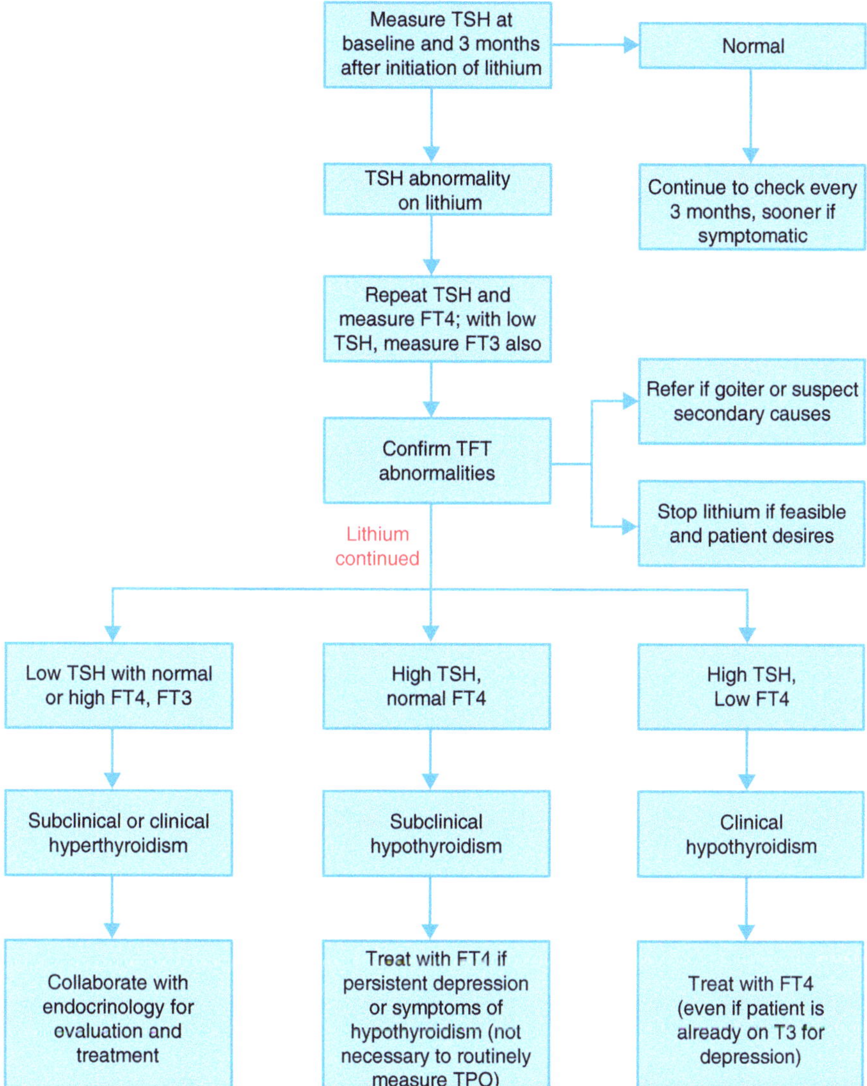

References

1. Lazarus JH. Lithium and thyroid. Best Pract Res Clin Endocrinol Metab. 2009;23(6):723–33.
2. McKnight RF, Adida M, Budge K, Stockton S, Goodwin GM, Geddes JR. Lithium toxicity profile: a systematic review and meta-analysis. Lancet. 2012;379(9817):721–8.
3. Bou Khalil R, Richa S. Thyroid adverse effects of psychotropic drugs: a review. Clin Neuropharmacol. 2011;34(6):248–55.

4. Escobar-Morreale HF, Botella-Carretero JI, Escobar del Rey F, Morreale de Escobar G. REVIEW: Treatment of hypothyroidism with combinations of levothyroxine plus liothyronine. J Clin Endocrinol Metab. 2005;90(8):4946–54.
5. Cooke RG, Joffe RT, Levitt AJ. T3 augmentation of antidepressant treatment in T4-replaced thyroid patients. J Clin Psychiatry. 1992;53(1):16–8.

Chapter 14
Hypercalcemia

Hypercalcemia is elevated serum calcium level >10.2 mg/dL. It is usually due to elevation in ionized free calcium but can be due to increased protein bound calcium seen in hyperalbuminemia.

Pathology

Calcium metabolism is regulated by parathyroid hormone (PTH) and vitamin D. Vitamin D increases intestinal absorption of calcium. PTH increases serum calcium by enhancing reabsorption by the renal tubule and mobilizing calcium stores from bone. It also stimulates conversion of vitamin D to its active metabolite. Low calcium levels cause a feedback increase in PTH secretion.

Etiology

The most common causes of elevated serum calcium are primary hyperparathyroidism and malignancy-related bone resorption. It can also be seen in hypervitaminosis D that results from excess ingestion of vitamin D. Primary hyperparathyroidism refers to an elevated PTH due to increased endogenous production from the parathyroid glands. Some medications, including lithium, cause hypercalcemia by inducing primary hyperparathyroidism.

© Springer International Publishing AG 2017
A. Annamalai, *Medical Management of Psychotropic Side Effects*,
DOI 10.1007/978-3-319-51026-2_14

Psychotropic Medications and Hypercalcemia

Lithium changes the receptor set point for calcium sensing in parathyroid cells leading to increased PTH secretion and hypercalcemia. Lithium also has some direct effects on bone metabolism. Elevated levels are seen in almost 80% people in the few weeks after lithium administration but most remain within the normal range and are not clinically significant. In about 10% patients, long-term treatment leads to elevation of serum calcium beyond the normal range [1]. This usually occurs after many years of lithium treatment. Lithium seems to cause hyperplastic parathyroid disease though in many cases, parathyroid adenomas have been found [2]. The latter may represent an unmasking of preexisting clinically insignificant parathyroid adenomas.

If lithium is stopped, serum calcium levels return to normal in most but not all cases. In these patients, surgery to remove the hyperplastic parathyroid tissue may be necessary.

> *Lithium raises calcium and PTH levels to clinically significant levels in 10% patients.*

Clinical Features

Hypercalcemia is often asymptomatic. Possible clinical manifestations are neuropsychiatric disturbances (depression, cognitive dysfunction), gastric symptoms (anorexia, constipation), polyuria, nephrolithiasis, muscle weakness.

> *Hypercalcemia is often asymptomatic; symptoms when present are nonspecific.*

Diagnosis

Serum calcium is usually in the 10–12 mg/dL range in primary hyperparathyroidism, including in lithium-induced hyperparathyroidism. Higher levels are likely to be due to non-PTH-mediated causes and require testing for vitamin D toxicity, sarcoidosis, malignancy, etc.

The hypercalcemia can be confirmed by measuring an ionized calcium level but this is generally not necessary if the serum albumin is normal. A serum PTH is useful to differentiate PTH-mediated hypercalcemia from other causes of hypercalcemia. A high PTH indicates hyperparathyroidism rather than malignancy or hypervitaminosis D. However, the PTH (or other lab tests) cannot differentiate lithium-induced hyperparathyroidism from endogenous primary hyperparathyroidism. It is to be noted that in patients with chronic kidney disease, though PTH is high, calcium is usually low. The hyperparathyroidism in this case is due to hypocalcemia-induced PTH secretion. In later stages of kidney disease, calcium levels may also rise with exogenous replacement.

> ***In lithium-induced hyperparathyroidism both PTH and calcium are high. If calcium is high and PTH is low, other causes should be sought.***

Management

Serum calcium should be checked at baseline before starting lithium and then at regular intervals during treatment. If calcium rises, PTH can be measured to rule out other causes of hypercalcemia. If there is a mild rise in serum calcium up to 11 mg/dL and patient is asymptomatic, lithium can be continued. If serum calcium rises >11 mg/dL there should be consideration for stopping lithium. If serum calcium rises >12 mg/dL, lithium should be stopped. At any stage, lithium should be stopped if patient is symptomatic. Since lithium can induce parathyroid hyperplasia, calcium level should be rechecked 4–6 weeks after stopping lithium. If the serum calcium remains high, patient should be referred for evaluation for surgical resection and to rule out other etiologies. If partial parathyroid resection is done and lithium is continued, there is a high chance of recurrence of the hyperparathyroidism.

Cinacalcet is a calcimimetic agent that enhances calcium receptor sensitivity and reduces PTH secretion and consequently calcium levels. Bisphosphonates inhibit bone resorption and are used in people with untreated hyperparathyroidism. Both cinacalcet and bisphosphonates are used in hyperparathyroidism treatment but have limited utility in lithium-induced parathyroid disease.

> ***If serum calcium levels rise >11 mg/day during lithium treatment, medication switch should be considered as rising calcium levels may indicate development of parathyroid hyperplasia.***
>
> ***Endocrinology consult is warranted if calcium level is equivocal and lithium is important for psychiatric symptoms or hyperparathyroidism does not reverse after stopping lithium.***

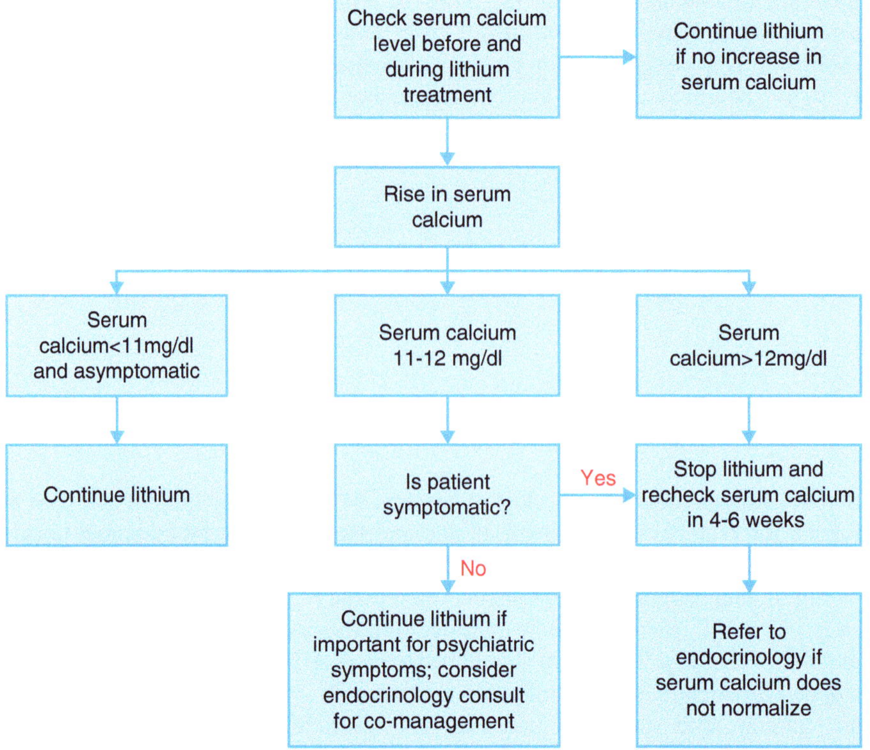

References

1. Mallette LE, Eichhorn E. Effects of lithium carbonate on human calcium metabolism. Arch Intern Med. 1986;146(4):770–6.
2. Skandarajah AR, Palazzo FF, Henry JF. Lithium-associated hyperparathyroidism: surgical strategies in the era of minimally invasive parathyroidectomy. World J Surg. 2011;35(11): 2432–9.

Section V
Kidney and Electrolytes

Chapter 15
Diabetes Insipidus

Diabetes insipidus (DI) is a syndrome characterized by abnormally large volumes of dilute urine due to decreased secretion or action of antidiuretic hormone (ADH). The polyuria is associated with increased thirst leading to a commensurate increase in fluid intake, polydipsia.

Pathology

Antidiuretic hormone (ADH) or vasopressin is synthesized in the hypothalamus and secreted from the posterior lobe of the pituitary gland. The normal action of ADH on the renal tubules is to promote water reabsorption and prevent diuresis. Deficiency of ADH secretion or resistance to ADH action on renal tubules causes excessive water excretion and a syndrome of diabetes insipidus.

Etiology

Central diabetes insipidus is caused by deficiency of ADH secretion due to genetic abnormalities or secondary to many central nervous system disorders.

Nephrogenic diabetes insipidus results from deficiencies in the action of ADH. Nephrogenic DI can result from inherited causes, but more commonly is secondary to systemic disorders or drugs. DI results when disorders or drugs disrupt the sensitivity of the kidneys to ADH and impair concentrating ability.

© Springer International Publishing AG 2017
A. Annamalai, *Medical Management of Psychotropic Side Effects*,
DOI 10.1007/978-3-319-51026-2_15

Psychotropic Medications and Diabetes Insipidus

Lithium is well known to cause nephrogenic DI. Lithium impairs the concentrating ability of the kidney by its action on the collecting tubule. Up to 54% patients on lithium show an impaired concentrating ability but a fewer proportion of people manifest overt polyuria [1]. With continued lithium treatment, it is estimated that about 20–40% people develop irreversible and overt polyuria that may be seen even years after lithium treatment [2]. Even though the defect in concentrating ability is initially reversible, after chronic lithium maintenance therapy, the tubular dysfunction can convert to irreversible polyuria. Renal concentrating deficit can start within weeks to months of treatment but irreversible polyuria usually takes many years to develop. The urinary concentrating ability improves immediately after lithium discontinuation but does not return to baseline in all patients [3]. Persistent renal concentrating deficit is associated with duration of lithium use, total and maximum doses of lithium administered, and simultaneous use of antipsychotics. Recurrent episodes of lithium toxicity may predispose to DI.

DI may be a risk factor for developing chronic kidney disease though the latter is much less prevalent than DI.

Some cases of DI from clozapine have also been reported but far less frequently than lithium [4].

> ***Chronic lithium treatment can cause irreversible polyuria in up to 40% people; higher doses, longer duration of treatment, and recurrent episodes of lithium toxicity are risk factors.***

Clinical Features

Polyuria with large volumes of urine, even up to 20 L a day is the hallmark of DI. It is often associated with nocturia. Most people are able to compensate for the loss of fluids by an increased thirst response leading to polydipsia. Cognitively impaired individuals or elderly with dementia or those with poor access to water may develop volume depletion and resultant hypernatremia. Hypernatremia causes neurologic symptoms by water movement out of brain cells and resultant decrease in brain size. Initial symptoms are lethargy, weakness that can progress to twitching, seizures, and coma. Generally, severe symptoms do not develop unless serum sodium levels are above 150 meq/L.

> ***Polyuria and polydipsia are the primary symptoms; lethargy and more serious neurologic symptoms are seen if hypernatremia develops.***

Diagnosis

History can rule out other common disorders causing polyuria such as diabetes mellitus, acute urinary tract infections, and prostatic hypertrophy. Primary polydipsia should be considered as a cause of the polyuria. Determining if polyuria preceded the polydipsia may be useful to distinguish between DI and primary polydipsia.

Serum sodium is usually high in DI (>142 meq/L) and low in primary polydipsia (<137 meq/L). It can be a useful test to differentiate between the two conditions but the sodium level may be normal in both conditions.

Plasma osmolality is usually high normal but not higher than the normal range (295 mOsm) in DI because if the thirst mechanism is intact, then there is more water intake to compensate and reset the plasma osmolality. Similarly, in primary polydipsia, the plasma osmolality is low normal but not lower than 275 mOsm since water excretion compensates and resets the osmolality.

Urine osmolality is low in nephrogenic DI, usually <300 mOsm/kg. If urine osmolality is >600 mOsm/kg, it virtually rules out DI. In primary polydipsia, the urine osmolality is very low, usually <100 mOsm/kg as the kidney is actively excreting the excess water.

Serum sodium should be checked. Serum osmolality and urine osmolality can be tested for diagnostic clarification and to differentiate from primary polydipsia but as seen earlier, they may not be definitive.

Fluid deprivation test is the definitive test to diagnose nephrogenic DI and differentiate between that and primary polydipsia. However, the performance of this test is impractical in a behavioral health care setting and requires referral to an endocrinologist or nephrologist if diagnostic certainty is important for management.

> ***Serum sodium should be checked in patients on lithium with symptoms of polyuria and polydipsia; serum and urine osmolality are additional tests that may provide diagnostic clarity.***

Management

Maintaining lowest effective clinical dose of lithium and avoiding episodes of lithium toxicity can reduce the risk of developing polyuria. The risk of DI should be discussed with the patient before initiation of lithium. Renal concentrating deficit occurs before overt polyuria but there is no reliable way to measure this and no routine lab testing is recommended.

If polyuria occurs, lithium should be adjusted to lower therapeutic ranges and changed to single daily dose with a long-acting formulation. If polyuria persists, stopping lithium should be a consideration since there is a risk of conversion from a reversible to an irreversible renal concentrating deficit. It is not easy to pinpoint at what stage the polyuria becomes irreversible. There is unfortunately no reliable mechanism to predict which patients will develop irreversible polyuria.

If lithium is considered essential for the patient, then thiazide diuretics or amiloride can be considered. Diuretics act by decreasing extracellular fluid volume, promoting water resorption in the proximal tubule resulting in less water at the distal tubule where the deficit is present. Amiloride is preferable as it may also have an effect on preventing lithium uptake by the tubular cell. Either medication should preferably be instituted in concert with a nephrologist.

If primary polydipsia is suspected, mainstay of treatment is eliminating thirst-inducing medications and education on restricting fluid intake (see also Chapter 16). If the diagnosis is uncertain, it is reasonable to withhold lithium as a diagnostic trial and evaluate for persistence of symptoms.

No routine lab monitoring is required in asymptomatic patients.

If polyuria occurs, lithium dose should be reduced and changed to long-acting formulation; serum sodium and other lab testing can be done for diagnostic clarity.

If polyuria persists and nephrogenic DI is the likely cause, lithium should be stopped; if clinically necessary, diuretic therapy can be considered in conjunction with nephrology.

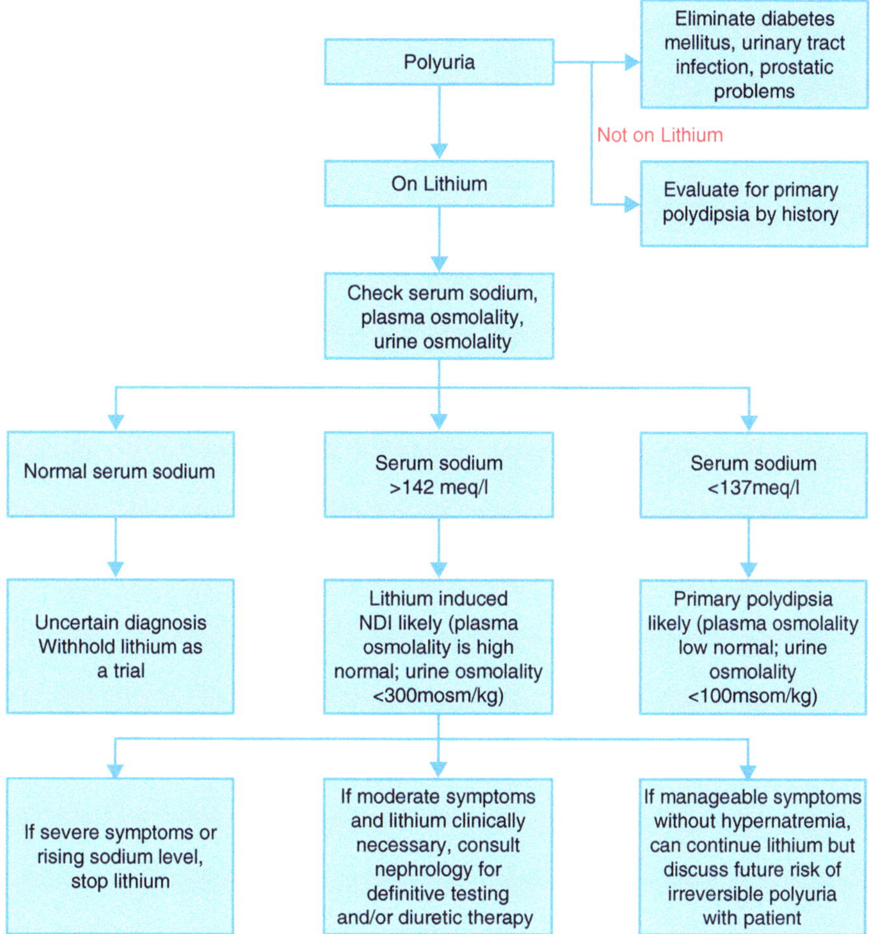

References

1. Boton R, Gaviria M, Batlle DC. Prevalence, pathogenesis, and treatment of renal dysfunction associated with chronic lithium therapy. Am J Kidney Dis. 1987;10(5):329–45.
2. Stone KA. Lithium-induced nephrogenic diabetes insipidus. J Am Board Fam Pract. 1999; 12(1):43–7.
3. Bucht G, Wahlin A. Renal concentrating capacity in long-term lithium treatment and after withdrawal of lithium. Acta Med Scand. 1980;207(4):309–14.
4. Bendz H, Aurell M. Drug-induced diabetes insipidus: incidence, prevention and management. Drug Saf. 1999;21(6):449–56.

Chapter 16
Hyponatremia

Hyponatremia represents a state of excess total body water in relation to body sodium content. The serum sodium level is <135 meq/L.

Pathology

Volume status is critical in determining the sodium balance and etiology of low serum sodium levels. In states of volume depletion, there is loss of both sodium and water but the primary sodium loss exceeds the total body water loss. In states of volume excess such as edematous states, the total body water is increased in relation to the total body sodium. Though there is an excess of extracellular fluid, the effective plasma volume is reduced. And this causes secretion of antidiuretic hormone (ADH) and further lowering of the sodium level. In some conditions, as with central nervous system disorders, ADH is secreted inappropriately, causing water retention and a secondary reduction in serum sodium levels.

Medications cause release of ADH resulting in a state similar to syndrome of inappropriate ADH (SIADH). Some of the effect on sodium is also postulated to be a change in renal collecting tubule response to ADH.

Etiology

Primary polydipsia, a condition where there is excess water consumption, is common in patients with mental illness. Hyponatremia occurs as the water consumption exceeds the capacity of the kidney to excrete free water, which is either because the water consumption is excessively high or there is a defect in the excretory capacity of the kidney.

Many medications, including some psychotropic agents, cause an SIADH like state.

© Springer International Publishing AG 2017

A. Annamalai, *Medical Management of Psychotropic Side Effects*,

DOI 10.1007/978-3-319-51026-2_16

Pseudohyponatremia is a condition where the serum sodium and serum osmolality are both normal but serum sodium is artificially low due to presence of other solutes in blood such as glucose or lipids.

See table in appendix for common etiologies of hyponatremia with corresponding volume status with each condition.

Psychotropic Medications and Hyponatremia

Carbamazepine and oxcarbazepine are two agents associated with the highest prevalence of hyponatremia (15% and 30%, respectively). Though prevalence is high, very low sodium levels <130 meq/L occur only at a prevalence of 1.29% in oxcarbazepine and 0.1% with carbamazepine. Hyponatremia also occurs with other psychotropic agents [1]. The prevalence of hyponatremia with SSRIs and SNRIs is low (0.06% and 0.08%, respectively). Antipsychotics are rarely associated with hyponatremia, though some studies report a high prevalence [2]. Risk of hyponatremia increases if combined with other agents that reduce sodium level such as diuretics.

Hyponatremia from medications usually occurs early in treatment but can be seen later. There is no clear evidence that medication dose or serum levels have any correlation with the risk or degree of hyponatremia. Usually once the hyponatremia develops, it persists as long as the medication is continued. One clearly established risk factor is advanced age.

> ***Mild hyponatremia is associated with many psychotropic medications but sodium reduction <130 mmol/L is rare; effect on sodium usually occurs early in treatment.***

Clinical Features

Symptoms depend on both the severity and rapidity of decline in sodium levels. The symptoms are mainly neurological and related to the hyposmolality that accompanies hyponatremia causing increased movement of water into cells. Brain edema causes the neurologic symptoms.

The earliest signs of hyponatremia are nausea and malaise and may be seen in serum sodium levels less than 130 meq/L, but more likely below 125 meq/L. Headache, lethargy, obtundation, and eventually coma can occur when the serum sodium falls below 120 meq/L. These symptoms occur only when the hyponatremia develops over 24 h or so. When the serum sodium falls more slowly, the brain cells compensate by creating a gradient for the extracellular fluid out of the brain into the cerebrospinal fluid. In chronic hyponatremia, symptoms are generally nonspecific such as nausea, malaise, dizziness, forgetfulness.

> ***Clinical manifestations of hyponatremia usually occur only when it develops rapidly in less than 24 h and when sodium level is <125 meq/L.***

Diagnosis

Hyponatremia is a consideration in patients complaining of nausea or malaise when there is a suspicion of either polydipsia or patient is on psychotropic medications. A history will help distinguish between medication-related hyponatremia and excess fluid consumption.

Additional laboratory tests are not necessary but urine osmolality can help differentiate hyponatremia secondary to primary polydipsia from other causes of hyponatremia, including medications. Urine osmolality normally ranges from 300 to 1200 mOsm/kg. In primary polydipsia, the response to excess water consumption is excretion of a very dilute urine with osmolality <100 mOsm/kg and specific gravity ≤1.003. With most other causes of hyponatremia, there is persistent or inappropriate ADH release resulting in a urine osmolality >300 mOsm/kg.

Serum osmolality is low in both primary polydipsia and medication-induced hyponatremia. In fact, it is low in all causes of hyponatremia except pseudohyponatremia. Normal serum osmolality has a narrow range from 275 to 290 mOsm/kg.

History is generally sufficient to differentiate primary polydipsia from other etiologies causing hyponatremia; if desired, urine osmolality can be measured to confirm the diagnosis.

Management

If the patient has sodium <125 meq/L that is new onset or of unknown duration or sodium >125 meq/L with new symptoms, urgent intervention may be needed in the form of intravenous sodium chloride replacement. If hyponatremia develops slowly and serum sodium remains >125 meq/L in an asymptomatic patient, the cause should be established. Other etiologies such as acute gastroenteritis, diuretic therapy, cirrhosis, and kidney dysfunction should be considered.

If primary polydipsia is suspected or confirmed, the first step in treatment is water restriction. Attention should also be paid to medications that could be causing increased thirst such as anticholinergic agents. If water restriction is not feasible or it is inadequate for maintaining normal serum sodium levels, the sodium level should be monitored periodically. Monthly monitoring is usually sufficient for most people with serum sodium level >130 meq/L.

In patients on psychotropic medications that are suspected to cause the hyponatremia, the agent should be stopped unless clinically necessary. Even in chronic hyponatremia without overt symptoms there may be subtle neurologic signs such as minor gait imbalance or memory loss. Treatment of mild hyponatremia due to medications may be resolved by water restriction.

The extent of fluid restriction depends on severity of hyponatremia. Reducing fluid intake to less than 50% of usual recommended intake (800–1000 mL/day) may be required if serum sodium is lower than 125 meq/L.

In patients with chronic hyponatremia due to unchangeable causes, demeclocycline, a tetracycline derivative that increases ADH resistance is used. Generally there is no role for this in drug-induced hyponatremia as it is preferable to stop the causative agent. In the rare circumstance where the offending psychotropic agent is considered essential, demeclocycline can be considered in consultation with a nephrologist [3].

An emergency room evaluation is warranted for sodium <125 meq/L, rapid reduction to sodium <130 meq/L, and any sodium level with new symptoms.

Fluid restriction is the mainstay of treatment in hyponatremia from primary polydipsia.

Mild psychotropic-induced hyponatremia may not need any intervention.

Stopping the medication is the strategy of choice in moderate to severe hyponatremia unless the offending medication is absolutely necessary.

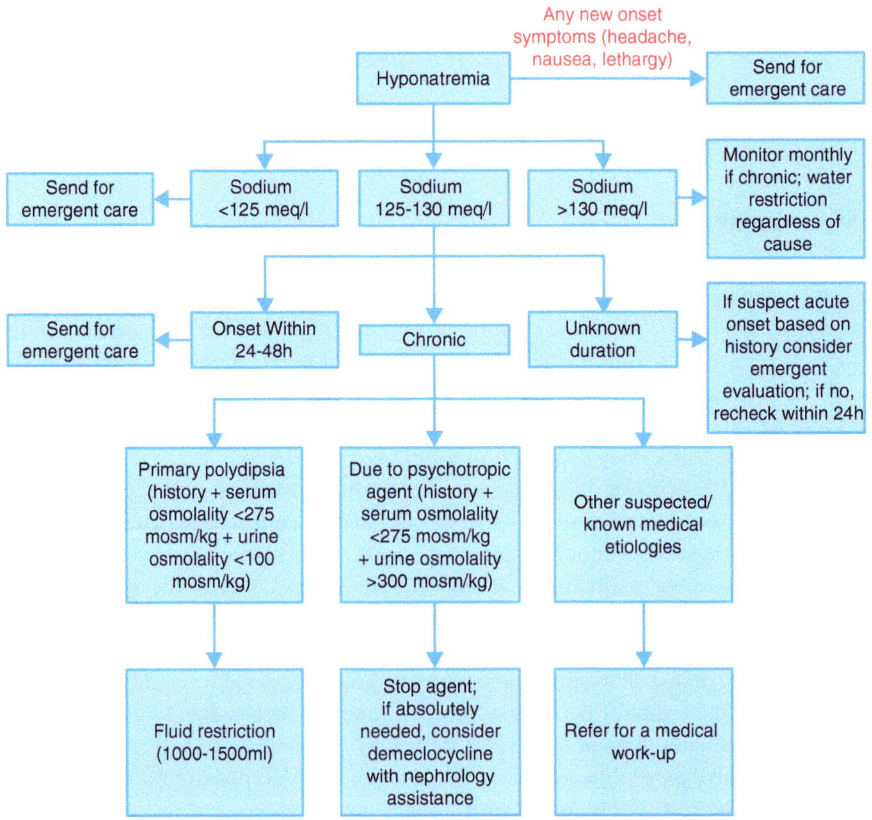

Appendix: Common Etiologies of Hyponatremia

Volume status	Clinical conditions
Hypovolemic (state of volume depletion where primary sodium loss exceeds total body water loss)	Gastroenteritis (loss of sodium with replacement by water)
	Acute tubular necrosis (salt losing nephropathy)
	Diuretics, e.g., thiazides (increase sodium excretion)
	Postobstructive diuresis (increased sodium excretion)
Hypervolemic (decreased circulating volume but excess extracellular fluid with resultant total body water retention)	Heart failure
	Cirrhosis
	Nephrotic syndrome
Euvolemic (from increased total body water and secondary dilutional reduction in sodium)	SIADH (inappropriate ADH release in central nervous system disorders, malignancies, recent surgery, Addisons disease, hypothyroidism)
	Medications
	Pesudohyponatremia (normal osmolality but spurious low sodium level due to hyperlipidemia, hyperglycemia, hyperproteinemia)

References

1. Letmaier M, Painold A, Holl AK, Vergin H, Engel R, Konstantinidis A, et al. Hyponatraemia during psychopharmacological treatment: results of a drug surveillance programme. Int J Neuropsychopharmacol. 2012;15(6):739–48.
2. Serrano A, Rangel N, Carrizo E, Uzcátegui E, Sandia I, Zabala A, et al. Safety of long-term clozapine administration. Frequency of cardiomyopathy and hyponatraemia: two cross-sectional, naturalistic studies. Aust N Z J Psychiatry. 2014;48(2):183–92.
3. Spigset O, Hedenmalm K. Hyponatraemia and the syndrome of inappropriate antidiuretic hormone secretion (SIADH) induced by psychotropic drugs. Drug Saf. 1995;12(3):209–25.

Chapter 17
Chronic Kidney Disease

Chronic kidney disease (CKD) is a progressive loss of renal function, lasting at least 3 months that can lead to irreversible end-stage renal failure.

Pathology

The normal kidney is able to maintain its function in the face of renal injury and overt abnormalities are not seen until at least 50% of filtration capacity is lost. Progressive renal damage can occur from glomerular disease, tubulointerstitial disease, or chronic obstructive pathology. Major effects of renal failure include electrolyte and volume imbalance, anemia, and bone disease.

Etiology

Common causes of CKD in the United States are hypertension and diabetes followed by glomerulonephritis. There are various immunologic, infectious, and vascular diseases as well as drugs that can cause CKD.

Psychotropic Medications and CKD

See Chapter 1 for recommendations on using psychotropic medications in preexisting renal disease. Following is a review of psychotropic-induced renal failure.

Among psychotropic medications, lithium is implicated in CKD. The exact magnitude of risk of CKD with lithium use is uncertain but is estimated to be small. There is a reduction of glomerular filtration rate (GFR), an estimate of kidney

© Springer International Publishing AG 2017

A. Annamalai, *Medical Management of Psychotropic Side Effects*,
DOI 10.1007/978-3-319-51026-2_17

function, over time with lithium. However, the absolute risk of end-stage failure is thought to be only about 0.5%, which is slightly higher than the general population [1]. Lithium's adverse effect on kidney function is mainly via interstitial injury and to a smaller extent, glomerular injury. Lithium causes renal tubular dysfunction and concentrating deficit earlier in treatment (see Chapter 15) but lithium-induced nephropathy results from chronic use.

Duration of lithium use is linked to risk of CKD. It is estimated that it takes 10–20 years for lithium-induced kidney damage to progress to kidney failure [2]. High lithium dosages are also thought to increase the risk. Dosing lithium multiple times during the day increases the risk compared to once-daily dosing. Episodes of lithium toxicity predispose to development of chronic renal failure. In addition to overdose, risks for nephrotoxicity include advanced age, other medications that affect renal function, other medical conditions that can cause CKD, decreased circulating volume, and diabetes insipidus that is also a side effect of lithium (see Chapter 15).

> ***Risk of CKD from lithium use is small.***
>
> ***Nephrotoxicity develops over long duration of use.***

Risk factors for lithium induced CKD

Duration of treatment
Higher lithium doses
Multiple times a day dosing
Multiple episodes of acute lithium toxicity
Concomitant long-term use of nephrotoxic drugs and presence of medical conditions that can cause nephrotoxicity

Clinical Features

Deteriorating renal function is usually asymptomatic until there is significant decline. An episode of acute renal injury may cause a state of uremia with symptoms of general malaise and nausea. Symptoms may result from complications of CKD, such as volume overload, electrolyte imbalance, bone disorders, elevated blood pressure, anemia, lipid abnormalities, sexual dysfunction.

> ***CKD is asymptomatic until later stages.***

Diagnosis

There is no mechanism to definitively assess for lithium as the cause of kidney disease in an individual with coexisting morbidities. It is thus important to assess renal function at baseline and monitor periodically.

GFR is considered the best index of renal function. It declines with progressive kidney disease though the magnitude of decline does not always correlate with the extent of kidney damage. The gold standard for GFR measurement is by using clearance of exogenous markers such as inulin. A 24-h creatinine clearance is also used as a proxy for GFR. In clinical practice, GFR is estimated by prediction equations based on serum creatinine level. The prediction equations take into account age, race, and gender variations. Most laboratories perform this calculation and report this as part of renal function. These predictions are not without pitfalls but are convenient tools to use in routine practice. GFR <60 mL/min is considered the beginning of CKD and a GFR<15 mL/min is end-stage renal disease (ESRD).

Serum creatinine, which is used in calculating GFR, can independently be used as a gross marker of kidney function. However, diet, hydration status, excessive exercise, and extremes of weight affect serum creatinine. Also creatinine lags behind GFR in initial stages of CKD.

Excretion of albumin in urine is also considered a marker of kidney function and long-term prognosis. Albuminuria is used in staging of CKD. Given that a 24-h urine albumin measurement is impractical in many situations, a spot urine albumin creatinine ratio (ACR) is used.

For monitoring kidney function on lithium, GFR can be used as a marker. If the laboratory is unable to report an estimated GFR, practitioners can use online calculators that are available. Serum creatinine can also be used as a gross marker. Some experts recommend monitoring ACR for patients on lithium [3]. This is still under debate as lithium causes minimal glomerular injury and proteinuria.

Chronic interstitial injury can also cause abnormal red cells in the urine and red or white cell casts but this is generally not used in assessing lithium induced renal damage.

> ***Calculated GFR should be used to measure kidney function; serum creatinine can be used as a gross estimate.***

Management

GFR and serum creatinine should be measured at baseline. Lithium is not recommended for GFR <40 mL/min. At GFR > 40 <60 mL/min, it may be warranted if other options are limited. For GFR >60 mL/min, lithium can be initiated.

Renal function, along with electrolytes, should be monitored biweekly to monthly during lithium dose titration. For patients on stable lithium doses, it can be measured yearly or every 6 months for those with other risk factors for CKD. If renal function declines, lithium continuation will depend on the benefits of lithium for that particular patient and availability of alternatives. Stopping lithium halts the decline in renal function and is thought to improve it until a certain point. A GFR <40 mL/min is thought to be the CKD stage beyond which lithium-induced renal damage is irreversible and continues even if lithium is stopped [2].

Lithium should be stopped if GFR <40 mL/min and there is stage 4 CKD. For GFR <60 >40 mL/min, lithium should preferably be stopped.

Some experts suggest using proteinuria as an adjunctive test to GFR to aid in decision-making. It is recommended that lithium be stopped for any amount of proteinuria arising from lithium treatment.

When patient is on lithium avoid, is possible, routine use of thiazide diuretics, nonsteroidal anti-inflammatory drugs, and angiotensin-converting enzyme inhibitors. These agents can increase lithium levels and contribute to acute toxicity as well as chronic nephrotoxicity.

Lithium-induced kidney damage becomes irreversible at a certain stage, likely around GFR 40 mL/min.

Lithium can be initiated or continued at GFR>60 mL/min; it should not be used at <40 mL/min; at GFR<60 >40 mL/min, it is not recommended but may be used in consultation with a nephrologist for compelling indications.

Proteinuria may be used as an adjunctive test to measure kidney function on lithium.

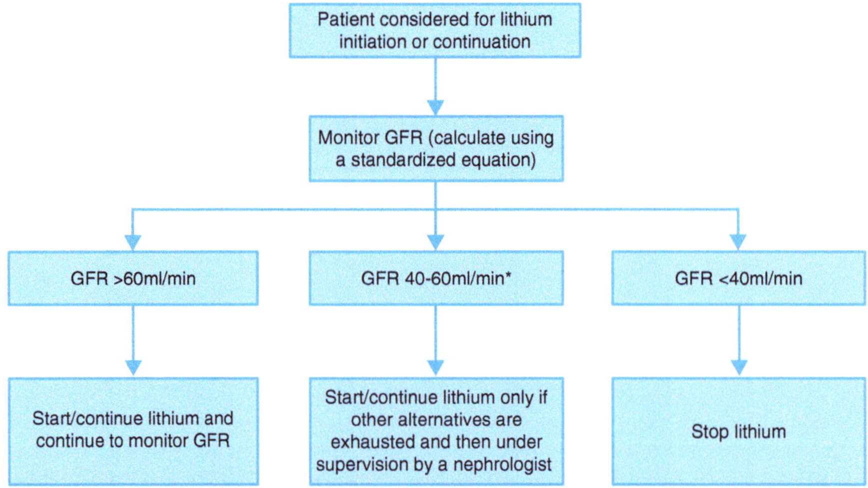

*May be useful to measure albumin creatinine ratio; if >30mg/mmol, stop lithium

References

1. McKnight RF, Adida M, Budge K, Stockton S, Goodwin GM, Geddes JR. Lithium toxicity profile: a systematic review and meta-analysis. Lancet. 2012;379(9817):721–8.
2. Oliveira JL, Silva Junior GB, Abreu KL, Rocha Nde A, Franco LF, Araujo SM, et al. Lithium nephrotoxicity. Rev Assoc Med Bras. 2010;56(5):600–6.
3. Kripalani M, Shawcross J, Reilly J, Main J. Lithium and chronic kidney disease. BMJ. 2009; 339:b2452.

Section VI
Genitourinary System

Chapter 18
Sexual Dysfunction

The prevalence of sexual dysfunction (SD), including mild, moderate, and severe dysfunction is estimated as high as 50% in both men and women and increases with age [1, 2].

Pathology

Disruption of sexual function can occur in any stage of the sexual cycle—desire, arousal, and ejaculatory phases. The most common SD in men is erectile dysfunction and can be caused by any factor that interferes with vascular and neural innervation to the penis. In women, the dysfunction can manifest in any phase including the desire/arousal phase.

Etiology

Each phase of sexual function is distinct and the particular dysfunction depends on the etiology. However, in clinical practice, patients present with dysfunction across phases and a clear distinction is not easily made.

Common causes of sexual dysfunction seen in practice are psychological problems (performance anxiety and relationship problems), recreational substances (tobacco, alcohol), obesity, diabetes, cardiovascular disease, liver or renal dysfunction, advanced age (postmenopausal, testosterone deficiency), and medications. Underlying depressive or anxiety disorders frequently cause sexual dysfunction.

The table in appendix lists examples of etiologies associated with each stage of sexual dysfunction.

© Springer International Publishing AG 2017

A. Annamalai, *Medical Management of Psychotropic Side Effects*,

DOI 10.1007/978-3-319-51026-2_18

Psychotropic Medications and Sexual Dysfunction

Medications may affect one sexual cycle phase more than others but typically the phases are interdependent and generally patients complain of side effects across phases. Men commonly complain of decreased libido and erectile dysfunction. Women commonly complain of decreased libido. Both men and women usually have decreased arousal and delayed orgasm, which may only be elicited on detailed questioning.

> *Even though medications may affect one sexual phase more than the other, generally patients present with dysfunction across phases.*

All three major neurotransmitters, dopamine, serotonin, noradrenaline, affect sexual function. Agents that affect dopamine and serotonin are more commonly implicated in SD.

Prevalence of psychotropic-related SD is highly variable [3] and unreliable as many studies do not differentiate from SD caused by the underlying illness; also many are based on self-reported SD, which is likely lower. SD is reported anywhere from 20 to 80% across studies, it is likely in the 30–50% range. It may be slightly more prevalent in men than women [4].

SD appears to be dose related. It occurs early in treatment. It is reversible upon stopping the medication though there are case reports of persistent SD post-SSRI treatment [5]. Tolerance to this side effect usually does not develop and it only rarely resolves with time if medication is continued.

> *Sexual dysfunction from psychotropic medications is dose related, occurs early in treatment, and usually reverses when medication is stopped.*

Rare side effects reported with psychotropic medications are priapism (trazodone, some antipsychotics), painful ejaculation (tricyclic antidepressants), and spontaneous orgasms (serotonergic antidepressants) [4]. Priapism is discussed in more detail in Chapter 45.

Antidepressants

While there are no reliable rates of SD between different classes of antidepressants, strongly serotonergic agents are associated with higher rates of SD. Activation of 5HT2 receptor is thought to impair sexual function while activation of 5-HT1A may enhance sexual function. There is some suggestion that men commonly experience decreased desire, ejaculatory dysfunction, and delayed orgasm whereas women experience decreased arousal. See table for likelihood of SD with different antidepressants based on available evidence.

Phosphodiesterase inhibitors (PDE-5i) have shown efficacy in improving ejaculatory function and orgasm in men and there is some evidence to suggest a positive effect in women also. The effect on libido is smaller. Bupropion as an adjunctive therapy has shown equivocal benefit. Many other pharmacological agents such as buspirone, stimulants, dopamine agonists, antihistamines, and plant extracts have been studied but show mixed or negative results [6].

Antidepressants and sexual dysfunction

High risk	SSRIs—paroxetine > sertraline > escitalopram > venlafaxine > desvenlafaxine > fluoxetine > fluvoxamine > citalopram > duloxetine
Moderate risk	Tricyclic antidepressants, monoamine oxidase inhibitors
Low likelihood	Mirtazapine, bupropion

Generally strongly serotonergic antidepressants are associated with higher rates of sexual dysfunction.

Antipsychotics

Prolactin elevation due to dopamine blockade is thought to be the predominant mechanism in antipsychotic-induced SD but anticholinergic and alpha-adrenergic antagonistic effects also contribute. Retrograde ejaculation is associated with antipsychotics that have alpha adrenergic antagonistic activity. More commonly, men experience ejaculatory dysfunction and both men and women experience orgasmic dysfunction. Evidence comparing rates of SD among different antipsychotics is lacking. See table for grading of antipsychotics based on limited evidence.

There is some evidence for efficacy of PDE-5i for treatment of antipsychotic-induced SD [7]. Dopamine agonists have also been suggested as potential adjuncts but there is little evidence to support this.

Antipsychotics and sexual dysfunction

High	Typical antipsychotics, risperidone
Moderate	Clozapine, olanzapine
Low	Quetiapine, ziprasidone, aripiprazole

> *Generally antipsychotics with potent dopaminergic blockade are more likely to cause sexual dysfunction though anticholinergic and antiadrenergic effects also contribute.*

Other Psychotropic Agents

Among mood stabilizers, valproate and carbamazepine are associated with SD. Lithium has not been consistently associated with SD. Lamotrigine is thought to enhance sexual function. Benzodiazepines cause smooth muscle relaxation and have the potential to affect different phases of sexual function but there is no consistent evidence that they affect sexual function.

Clinical Features

As mentioned earlier, patients generally complain of dysfunction across phases. So they may present with reduced libido (diminished sexual desire or decreased arousal) or orgasmic dysfunction (incomplete or delayed orgasm). Men may present with erectile dysfunction (inability to acquire or sustain an erection) or delayed ejaculation.

> *Patients usually complain of a range of sexual problems from reduced libido to orgasmic dysfunction.*

Diagnosis

Obtaining a sexual history both before and after starting psychotropic medications is key to establishing medications as the etiology of SD. Underlying psychiatric illness like depression and schizophrenia are thought to affect the sexual desire phase more than other phases [4]. However, the nature of the dysfunction is unfortunately not a reliable measure to distinguish between SD from psychiatric illness and medication-induced SD. Hence, it is extremely important to assess for any SD prior to initiating psychotropic medication. A systematic inquiry is sufficient and there is no need for routine use of rating scales.

> *It is extremely important to obtain a sexual history before initiating a psychotropic medication, as this is the only way to reliably distinguish psychotropic-induced dysfunction from other causes.*

Management

The first step is to rule out other etiologies. If any medical conditions are suspected, patient should be referred for cardiovascular risk modification, treatment of any spinal or pelvic pathology, or modification of any hormonal deficiency. Attention should be paid to effect of recreational drugs and psychological or relationship factors.

There is no need to measure testosterone routinely. However, if it is done for any reason, patient should be referred for possible hormone replacement only if testosterone level is low.

If SD is suspected to be from either antidepressant or antipsychotic agents, the first step is to reduce the dose since this side effect is dose related. If not feasible due to reasons of efficacy, a switch to another medication with lower risk of SD should be considered. With antidepressants, transient discontinuation is a consideration but has not been systematically studied. Similarly, taking daily antidepressant with a short half-life just after sexual activity has been suggested but there is no good evidence to support this.

If earlier measures fail or cannot be attempted, treatment with an additional agent is the next step. Among the PDE-5i agents, any agent can be used though sildenafil and tadalafil have been studied in antidepressant-induced SD and sildenafil has been studied in antipsychotic-induced SD. Bupropion can also be tried as an adjunctive agent for antidepressant-induced SD though the evidence is lower than for the PDE-5i agents. Buspirone can also be tried though evidence is even lower. Even though dopamine agonists have been suggested, especially for antipsychotic-induced SD, it is not a recommended strategy since evidence is minimal and there is potential for psychotic symptom exacerbation.

In the rare situation that adjunctive agents including PDE-5i are ineffective and the medication is necessary, a referral to urology can be considered for penile injectable agents or prostheses. However, there is no evidence to support this for medication-induced SD.

> *Dose reduction or switch to alternative medication should be the initial strategy.*
>
> *Bupropion or buspirone can be tried as adjunctive therapy in antidepressant-induced sexual dysfunction.*
>
> *Phosphodiesterase inhibitors have shown the most efficacy in psychotropic-induced sexual dysfunction.*

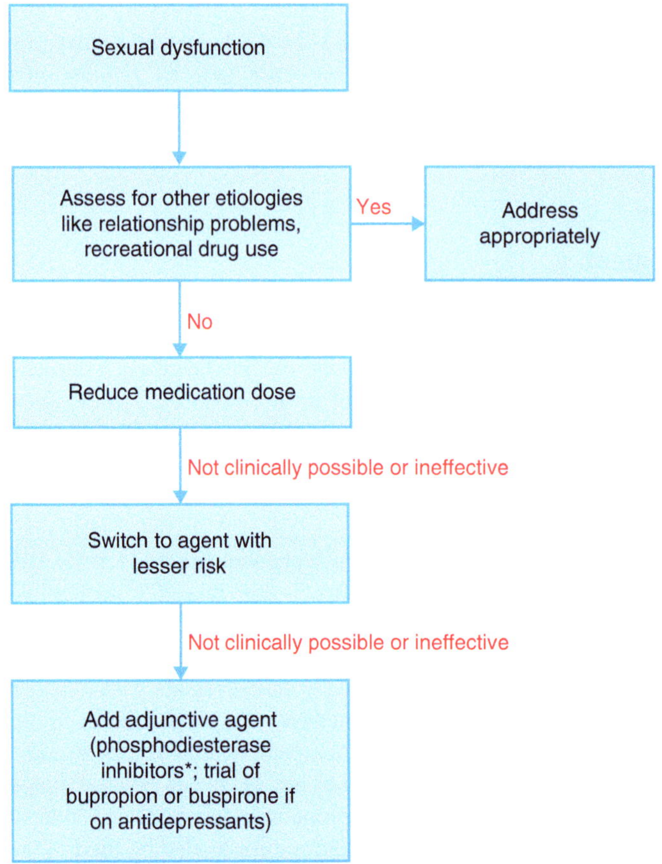

* Common side effect is facial flushing,headaches; contraindicated with nitrates; can be used cautiously in cardiac disease unless severe heart failure; rare reports of vision and hearing loss; dose may need to be lowered if using agents that inhibit CYP3A4

Appendix

Sexual dysfunction in males

Decreased libido (diminished desire or arousal)	Medications (e.g., antidepressants, opioids, antiandrogens)
	Depression
	Alcohol/recreational substances
	Testosterone deficiency
	Relationship problems
Erectile dysfunction (ED) (inability to acquire or sustain an erection)	Medications (e.g., antidepressants, antipsychotics, antihypertensives, antiandrogens, sympathetic blockers)
	Depression
	Obesity
	Smoking
	Diabetes
	Cardiovascular disease
	Spinal cord injury
	Pelvic trauma
	Testosterone deficiency and prolactin elevation
	Performance anxiety
Premature ejaculation (early ejaculation, may be associated with ED)	Performance anxiety/poor self-image (can be a factor in any stage)
	Vaginismus in partner
Delayed ejaculation, anorgasmia	Antidepressants
	Spinal or lower urinary tract surgery
Retrograde ejaculation	Antipsychotics
	Urinary sphincter abnormalities

Sexual dysfunction in females

Sexual interest/arousal disorder (diminished desire)	Medications (antidepressants, antihypertensives)
	Depression
	Alcohol use
	Hypoestrogenic states (high prolactin, menopause)
	Relationship problems
Orgasmic disorder (delay or absence of orgasm)	Medications (antidepressants)
	Depression
	Spinal cord injury
Vaginismus (pain or difficulty during penetration phase)	Anticholinergic medications (from vaginal dryness)
	Pelvic wall dysfunction (previous surgery or radiation)
	Endometriosis

References

1. Feldman HA, Goldstein I, Hatzichristou DG, Krane RJ, McKinlay JB. Impotence and its medical and psychosocial correlates: results of the Massachusetts Male Aging Study. J Urol. 1994;151(1):54–61.
2. Shifren JL, Monz BU, Russo PA, Segreti A, Johannes CB. Sexual problems and distress in United States women: prevalence and correlates. Obstet Gynecol. 2008;112(5):970–8.
3. Bella AJ, Shamloul R. Psychotropics and sexual dysfunction. Cent European J Urol. 2014;66(4):466–71.
4. Gitlin M. Sexual dysfunction with psychotropic drugs. Expert Opin Pharmacother. 2003;4(12):2259–69.
5. Csoka AB, Bahrick A, Mehtonen OP. Persistent sexual dysfunction after discontinuation of selective serotonin reuptake inhibitors. J Sex Med. 2008;5(1):227–33.
6. Taylor MJ, Rudkin L, Bullemor-Day P, Lubin J, Chukwujekwu C, Hawton K. Strategies for managing sexual dysfunction induced by antidepressant medication. Cochrane Database Syst Rev. 2013;5:CD003382.
7. Park YW, Kim Y, Lee JH. Antipsychotic-induced sexual dysfunction and its management. World J Mens Health. 2012;30(3):153–9.

Chapter 19
Urinary Incontinence and Retention

Urinary incontinence is the involuntary leakage of urine from the bladder due to lower urinary tract, pelvic, or neurologic abnormalities. It is seen in 15–20% of nonpregnant women and though less well studied in men, reported in up to 30% of men also.

Urinary retention is incomplete emptying of bladder and is defined as a postvoid residual volume of at least 50 mL. It is much more common in men.

Pathology

Normal micturition requires normal bladder muscle and sphincter function and an intact neural connection between the cerebral cortex and brainstem. Any disruption of bladder contraction, relaxation, or outlet function can result in incontinence.

Incontinence is classified into stress, urge, and overflow incontinence depending on the actual mechanism. The overflow incontinence results from incomplete bladder emptying.

Medications with anticholinergic, antihistaminic, analgesic effects may affect bladder function. The exact mechanism depends on the agent.

Etiology

In women, the likelihood of urinary incontinence increases with age and postmenopausal status due to changes in estrogen levels, detrusor activity, and urethral pressure. In men, with increasing age and prostate hypertrophy, risk for both urinary retention and incontinence increases.

In both women and men, obesity, neurologic disease, peripheral neuropathy, pelvic, or prostate surgery may cause or contribute to urinary problems. Urinary tract

© Springer International Publishing AG 2017

A. Annamalai, *Medical Management of Psychotropic Side Effects*,

DOI 10.1007/978-3-319-51026-2_19

infections (UTIs) and severe constipation with fecal impaction are temporary causes of incontinence, the former more common in women. Cognitive impairment and physical disability may limit capacity to use the bathroom appropriately and in time.

Caffeine and alcohol contribute to incontinence due to a diuretic effect and effect on bladder muscle contractility.

The etiology determines the type of incontinence and whether there is coexisting urinary retention. See appendix for common etiologies associated with urinary incontinence and urinary retention.

Psychotropic Medications and Urinary Symptoms

Overall incidence of psychotropic-induced urinary problems is low. The mechanism of urinary incontinence is mostly by alpha 1 adrenergic blockade causing decreased resistance of the urethral sphincter. Agents with alpha-adrenergic agonist activity also can experience incontinence due to increased urethral sphincter resistance and bladder overflow. Another important mechanism is anticholinergic action leading to decreased bladder activity and urinary retention with resultant overflow incontinence. Central dopaminergic blockade (causing detrusor muscle hyperactivity) and serotonergic inhibition (affecting parasympathetic bladder innervation) are also thought to play a role. Detrusor hyperactivity has been shown in urodynamic testing in people on atypical antipsychotics [1].

Among antipsychotics, clozapine is commonly implicated in urinary incontinence. It is also associated with enuresis. The two often occur together and while the mechanisms may be different for each, pharmacologic agents used for treatment are the same. Ephedrine has proved effective, postulated to be from an alpha-agonist effect [2]. There are case reports for successful resolution of incontinence with pseudoephedrine [3], oxybutynin, intranasal desmopressin [4], and aripiprazole [5]. However, aripiprazole itself is associated with enuresis, especially in children. Clozapine may also cause predominant symptoms of urinary retention with incomplete voiding.

Urinary incontinence can also occur with other antipsychotics [6]. Many typical antipsychotics including chlorpromazine, fluphenazine, and haloperidol also can cause urinary incontinence. The incontinence develops soon after the medication is initiated. It is dose related and the symptom resolves on stopping the medication.

Among antidepressants, tricyclic antidepressants can cause urinary retention due to their anticholinergic action. Selective serotonin reuptake inhibitors (SSRIs) also cause urinary incontinence in a small proportion of patients with sertraline carrying the highest risk [7]. It is thought to be due to potentiation of cholinergic neurotransmission and some dopamine blockade with sertraline. Venlafaxine may also cause this effect while duloxetine actually may improve incontinence. Benzodiazepines may contribute to urinary problems mainly due to sedative effect.

The table lists psychotropic medications commonly associated with urinary incontinence and retention.

Psychotropic agents most commonly associated with urinary symptoms

Tricyclic antidepressants (via anticholinergic action)
Antipsychotics—clozapine, olanzapine, risperidone (via multiple mechanisms)
Benzodiazepines (via sedation)
Alpha blockers—prazosin (via alpha adrenergic antagonism)

> ***Psychotropic medications can cause both urinary incontinence and retention; incontinence is more common. Urinary problems reverse on stopping the medication.***

Clinical Features

Patients with urge incontinence have an urge to void during bladder filling and experience some leakage before they can reach a bathroom. Patients with stress incontinence have some bladder leakage during activities that increase intra-abdominal pressure such as coughing, sneezing, and straining during bowel movements. Among younger women, stress incontinence is the more common type. In a majority of women, the incontinence is typically mixed type. Patients with overflow incontinence complain of incomplete voiding and leakage.

Patients on psychotropic medications usually present with mixed incontinence and possibly nocturnal enuresis. They may also present with more predominant features of urinary retention with anticholinergic side effects—weak urinary stream, intermittency, hesitancy, incomplete emptying, straining, and urgency. Men with BPH have similar symptoms, sometimes collectively called Lower Urinary Tract Symptoms (LUTS).

> ***Psychotropic-induced urinary incontinence typically presents as mixed type; medications with anticholinergic effects may cause symptoms similar to that associated with prostatic hypertrophy in men.***

Diagnosis

If patients complain of new-onset urinary incontinence, the type of incontinence should be determined by history. Clinicians should also assess for other symptoms such as urinary frequency and in men, LUTS. Voiding diaries may be helpful in determining if urinary frequency is related to intake of fluids including caffeine and alcohol. Easily treatable causes such as urinary tract infections and constipation can be usually ruled out by history. Specialists may consider postvoid residual measurement (<50 mL is adequate voiding and >200 mL is inadequate voiding) or other urodynamic measurements but these are neither necessary nor feasible in a psychiatric treatment setting.

> *A good history is generally sufficient to establish cause of urinary problems; additional testing is necessary only if diagnosis is uncertain or treatment is ineffective.*

Management

In a patient with urinary problems, common causes such as fluid, alcohol, caffeine consumption should be modified and nighttime intake limited if incontinence is present. Any easily treatable conditions such as severe constipation and UTI should be addressed appropriately. Patients who have recently been started on potentially causative medications like diuretics or antispasmodic agents should be referred to appropriate providers. If there are known causes such as previous spinal problems or pelvic surgery and there is new or worsening urinary incontinence, patients should be referred for further management.

For urinary incontinence, nonpharmacologic therapies are utilized as initial treatment, viz. bladder training (timed voiding to keep bladder volume low), pelvic floor exercises (Kegel exercises strengthen pelvic floor exercises), and mechanical devices (for predominant stress incontinence in women). Pelvic floor muscle training may be useful for symptoms of urinary retention also.

Pharmacologic treatment depends on specific etiology. Antimuscarinic agents (e.g., oxybutynin) are effective for urge incontinence while pessaries and other mechanical devices are more likely to help stress incontinence. However, since majority of patients present with mixed-type urinary incontinence, antimuscarinic agents are used as first-line medications. In postmenopausal women, topical estrogen reduces vaginal atrophy and improves incontinence.

In men with urinary retention and BPH, alpha blockers (e.g., terazosin) are first-line agents followed by 5-alpha reductase inhibitors (e.g., finasteride). Urinary retention is much less common in women and if it occurs, further urodynamic testing will likely be necessary to delineate the cause.

If patient is on a psychotropic medication that is causing urinary problems, incontinence is the more common presenting symptom. Nonpharmacological measures should be attempted first. Bladder training involves using the bathroom at specified intervals. Pelvic floor exercises can be tried in both women and men. If possible, the medication dose should be lowered as a trial.

If earlier measures do not alleviate incontinence, and it is severe and bothersome to patient, then medication should be switched to a different agent. In patients for whom the psychotropic medication is important for clinical benefit, as with clozapine, medications to treat urinary incontinence can be tried. Pseudoephedrine, ephedrine, intranasal desmopressin, or oxybutynin can be considered but patients should be monitored for side effects from these agents. Aripiprazole can be tried in the appropriate clinical situation. In some cases, urinary incontinence may resolve after the first 2–3 months [8] and it may be reasonable to wait before changing agents or using other treatments.

Patients with urinary retention may have bladder outlet obstruction and should be referred for further workup.

Nonpharmacological interventions should be tried in all cases of urinary incontinence.

Stopping causative medication will reverse the urinary side effects.

Antimuscarinic medications like oxybutynin can be tried for most types of incontinence including that from psychotropic medications.

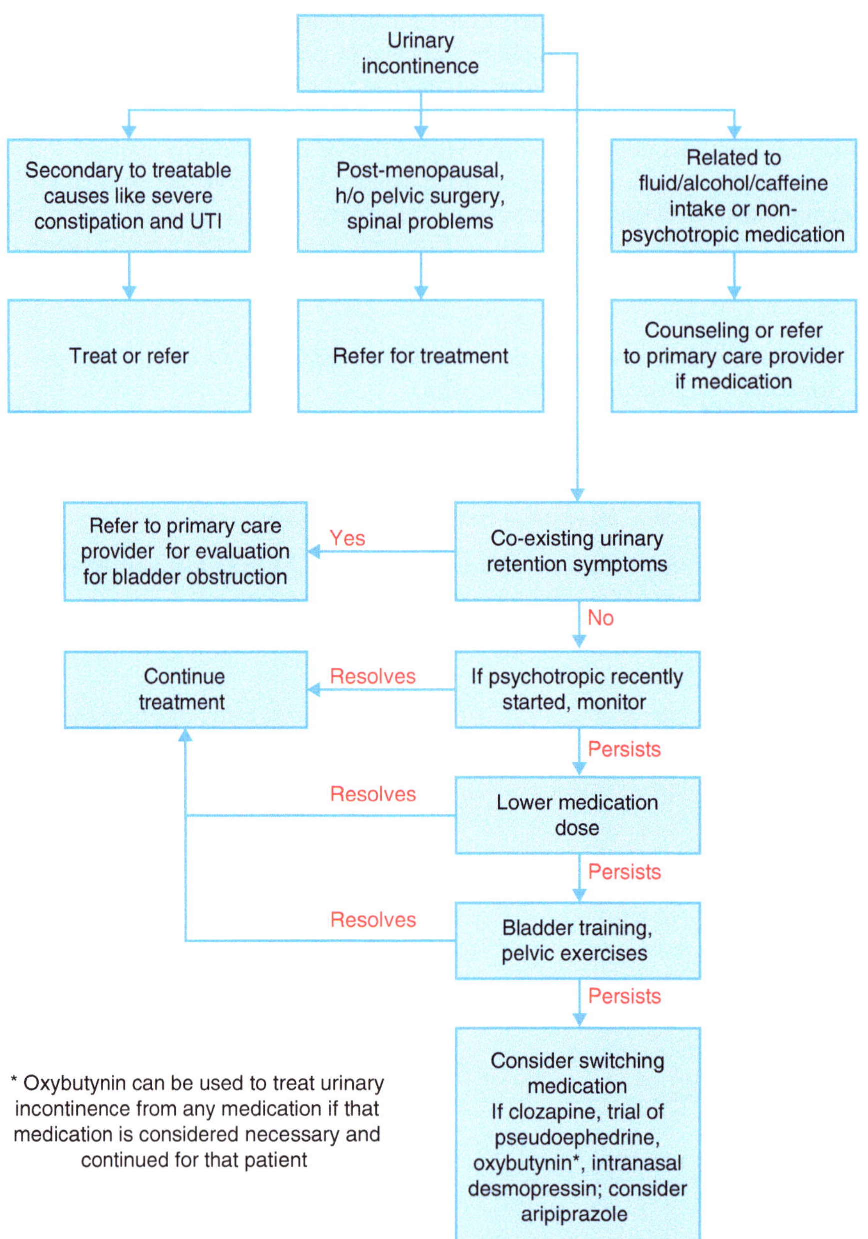
Urinary
incontinence

Secondary to treatable
causes like severe
constipation and UTI

Post-menopausal,
h/o pelvic surgery,
spinal problems

Related to
fluid/alcohol/caffeine
intake or non-
psychotropic medication

Treat or refer

Refer for treatment

Counseling or refer
to primary care provider
if medication

Refer to primary care
provider for evaluation
for bladder obstruction

Yes

Co-existing urinary
retention symptoms

No

Continue
treatment

Resolves

If psychotropic recently
started, monitor

Persists

Resolves

Lower medication
dose

Persists

Resolves

Bladder training,
pelvic exercises

Persists

Consider switching
medication
If clozapine, trial of
pseudoephedrine,
oxybutynin*, intranasal
desmopressin; consider
aripiprazole

* Oxybutynin can be used to treat urinary
incontinence from any medication if that
medication is considered necessary and
continued for that patient

Appendix

Etiologies of urinary incontinence in women

	Mechanism	Causes
Stress	Poor pelvic floor muscle support for urethra and bladder neck	Obesity
	Loss of normal urethral sphincter tone	Chronic cough
		Repeated vaginal deliveries
		Pelvic surgery
Urge	Bladder (detrusor) muscle hyperactivity	Neurologic disease or spinal cord injury
		Bladder abnormalities
Overflow	Decreased bladder (detrusor) muscle contractility	Age
		Low estrogenic state
		Peripheral neuropathy
		Multiple sclerosis
	Bladder outlet obstruction caused by external compression	Fibroid uterus
		Advanced pelvic prolapse
		Pelvic surgery

Etiologies of urinary incontinence in men

	Mechanism	Causes
Stress	Loss of normal urethral function	Prostate surgery
Urge	Bladder (detrusor) muscle hyperactivity	Neurologic disease or spinal cord injury
		Bladder abnormalities
Overflow	Decreased bladder (detrusor) muscle contractility	Age
		Peripheral neuropathy
	Bladder outlet obstruction	Benign prostatic hypertrophy

Selected modifiable etiologies of urinary incontinence in both men and women

Mechanism	Causes
Multiple mechanisms	Medications (antidepressants, antipsychotics, antihistamines, diuretics, antiparkinsonian drugs, antispasmodic agents)
Change in bladder contractility + diuretic effect	Alcohol
	Caffeine
Overflow due to external compression	Constipation
Due to increased frequency	Urinary tract infection

Common etiologies of urinary retention

	Mechanism	Causes
Men	Bladder outlet obstruction	Benign prostatic hypertrophy
		Prostate malignancy
Women	External compression	Uterine fibroids
		Pelvic organ prolapse
Men and women	Decreased bladder contractility	Age
		Peripheral neuropathy (e.g., diabetes mellitus)
		Many spinal cord disorders
		Medications
	Bladder outlet obstruction	Urethral stricture

References

1. Torre DL, Isgro S, Muscatello MR, Magno C, Melloni D, Meduri M. Urinary incontinence in schizophrenic patients treated with atypical antipsychotics: urodynamic findings and therapeutic perspectives. Int J Psychiatry Clin Pract. 2005;9(2):116–9.
2. Fuller MA, Borovicka MC, Jaskiw GE, Simon MR, Kwon K, Konicki PE. Clozapine-induced urinary incontinence: incidence and treatment with ephedrine. J Clin Psychiatry. 1996;57(11):514–8.
3. Hanes A, Lee Demler T, Lee C, Campos A. Pseudoephedrine for the treatment of clozapine-induced incontinence. Innov Clin Neurosci. 2013;10(4):33–5.
4. Lurie SN, Hosmer C. Oxybutynin and intranasal desmopressin for clozapine-induced urinary incontinence. J Clin Psychiatry. 1997;58(9):404.
5. Lee MJ, Kim CE. Use of aripiprazole in clozapine induced enuresis: report of two cases. J Korean Med Sci. 2010;25(2):333–5.
6. Harrison-Woolrych M, Skegg K, Ashton J, Herbison P, Skegg DC. Nocturnal enuresis in patients taking clozapine, risperidone, olanzapine and quetiapine: comparative cohort study. Br J Psychiatry. 2011;199(2):140–4.
7. Movig KL, Leufkens HG, Belitser SV, Lenderink AW, Egberts AC. Selective serotonin reuptake inhibitor-induced urinary incontinence. Pharmacoepidemiol Drug Saf. 2002;11(4):271–9.
8. Warner JP, Harvey CA, Barnes TR. Clozapine and urinary incontinence. Int Clin Psychopharmacol. 1994;9(3):207–9.

Section VII
Oral and Gastrointestinal System

Chapter 20
Hepatitis

Hepatitis is inflammation of the liver and detected usually by abnormal labs. Though liver function tests (LFTs) are a commonly used term for all tests related to the liver, some tests measure liver function and some measure biochemical health. Abnormalities in liver biochemistry do not necessarily reflect a defect in function.

Pathology

Liver disease can be broadly classified into hepatocellular injury and cholestatic disease that results from biliary disease or obstruction. The following tests are typically performed in labs as a test of liver health.

Lab tests to measure liver health

Test	Significance/cause of abnormality
Alanine aminotransferase (ALT)	Hepatic cell inflammation
Aspartate aminotransferase (AST)	Hepatic cell inflammation
Alkaline phosphatase (AP)	Mainly cholestasis from biliary obstruction; hepatic injury
Gamma glutamyl transpeptidase (GGT)	Cholestasis from biliary obstruction
Serum bilirubin	Both liver and biliary disease; hemolysis
Serum albumin	Liver synthetic function abnormality; kidney disease; malnutrition
Prothrombin test	Liver synthetic function; other bleeding and clotting disorders

© Springer International Publishing AG 2017   147
A. Annamalai, *Medical Management of Psychotropic Side Effects*,
DOI 10.1007/978-3-319-51026-2_20

Etiology

The most common causes for elevation in liver enzymes are listed as follows. Medications can cause both hepatocellular and cholestatic injury. Many medications can cause mild to modest hepatitis but only a few cause frank liver failure. A notable example is acetaminophen at high doses.

Most common causes of hepatic disease

Viral hepatitis
Alcoholic liver disease
Nonalcoholic fatty liver disease
Medication reaction

Other less common disease processes causing liver dysfunction include hemochromatosis (disorder of iron storage), Wilson disease (impaired cellular copper transport), autoimmune disease, alpha-1-antitrypsin deficiency (extra-pulmonary manifestation), and thyroid disorders. Some causes of biliary disease are Gilbert syndrome, hemolytic anemias, primary biliary cirrhosis, primary sclerosing chlolangitis, and other causes of bile duct obstruction.

Psychotropic Medications and Hepatitis

Psychotropic medications usually act by injury to hepatic cells though a cholestatic mechanism is implicated with some medications. The mechanism is metabolic or immune mediated. Some medications cause liver abnormalities by causing weight gain and subsequent fatty liver disease. Two psychotropic medications commonly known to cause liver injury are valproate (microvesicular steatosis is seen in liver cells) and carbamazepine (the liver toxicity appears to be part of a systemic hypersensitivity syndrome).

> *Psychotropic medications usually cause hepatic cell injury via a metabolic process or immune-mediated reaction; a cholestatic injury is less commonly implicated.*

Generally, the liver enzymes (usually transaminases) rise in the first 3–6 months of treatment. Mild hepatitis is seen in up to 30% patients on antipsychotics [1, 2]. Clinically significant elevations that require the medication to be discontinued occur in less than 5% cases. The prevalence of transaminase elevation with antidepressants, including clinically significant elevations, is less than 3% [3].

Naltrexone is generally safe to use in patients with preexisting liver disease. Though some studies suggest rise in transaminases up to 50%, clinically significant elevation occurs only in 1% patients [4].

Clinically significant elevation is considered rise of transaminases to at least more than two times normal or presence of clinical symptoms. Liver enzymes generally return to normal when the medication is stopped. Even when medication is continued, the enzyme abnormality has been reported to resolve in approximately 50% cases of antipsychotics [1]. Age and polypharmacy are risk factors to develop hepatic injury. Preexisting liver disease may predispose to developing hepatitis though evidence is unclear on this. Liver injury is generally considered to be independent of medication dose.

> ***Rise in transaminases usually occurs in first 3–6 months of treatment and can occur even at low doses; elevation that is more than two times normal is considered clinically significant.***

See table for summary of risk propensity of different psychotropic agents.

Psychotropic medications and risk of hepatocellular injury[a]

Class	Higher risk	Low risk	Rare/none
Mood stabilizers, (High: 10%, Low: <1%)	Valproate, carbamazepine	Lamotrigine, oxcarbazepine	Lithium
Antipsychotics (High: About 30%, Low: About 5%)	Chlorpromazine, olanzapine, clozapine	Perphenazine, fluphenazine, haloperidol, risperidone	Quetiapine, ziprasidone, aripiprazole
Antidepressants (High: 1–3%, Low: 0.3–1%)	Monoamine oxidase inhibitors (MAOIs), tricyclic antidepressants (TCAs), duloxetine, mirtazapine	Bupropion, sertraline, venlafaxine, fluoxetine	Citalopram, escitalopram, fluvoxamine
Antianxiety agents	–	–	Benzodiazepines, buspirone

[a]The percentage risk in this table refers to any elevation of transaminases; the risk of clinically significant elevations is lower than indicated here

Acute liver failure is rare and prevalence is based mainly on case reports. The psychotropic agents most commonly linked with acute hepatic failure are valproate, carbamazepine, and chlorpromazine. Transaminase elevation is not a good predictor of future liver failure. The acute failure can occur after a gradual rise or can be idiosyncratic and occur suddenly. Information on individual agents can be found at livertox.nlm.nih.gov.

> ***Among psychotropic agents, valproate, carbamazepine, and chlorpromazine are implicated in acute hepatic failure.***
>
> ***Transaminase elevation is not a good predictor of acute hepatic failure.***

Hyperammonemia

Ammonia elevation is normally seen in liver disease. However, valproate is known to cause elevated ammonia in the absence of liver disease. It occurs even at therapeutic doses and normal serum levels of valproate [5]. It usually occurs within a few days of starting the medication and patients may present with signs of encephalopathy. The ammonia level is only slightly elevated in some cases [6]. Stopping the medication rapidly reverses the ammonia levels and any clinical symptoms. A lack of carnitine is thought to contribute to the mechanism of hyperammonemia [6]. Levocarnitine is an effective and safe treatment in cases of acute hyperammonemia.

Cases of carbamazepine-induced hyperammonemia are also reported. Mechanism is speculated as similar to that of valproate.

> ***Ammonia elevation can occur with valproate therapy even without signs of liver injury; it can occur even at normal therapeutic serum levels.***

Clinical Features

The majority of people with elevated transaminases are asymptomatic. Some patients may present with nonspecific symptoms of anorexia, nausea, fatigue, and abdominal pain. With significant transaminase elevation, there may be manifestations of liver damage like jaundice and dark urine. If ammonia is high or there is severe hepatotoxicity, mental status changes may be seen.

> ***Patients with medication-induced transaminase elevation are usually asymptomatic as the liver injury is mild in most cases.***

Diagnosis

In general, transaminases (AST, ALT) are the enzymes more likely to be affected by psychotropic medications. With more severe hepatic injury, other enzymes will also rise. If nonmedication causes are suspected, the pattern of enzyme elevation can be used to distinguish between hepatic and cholestatic etiologies.

In alcoholic hepatitis, AST is typically higher than ALT, often in the 2:1 ratio. AST is usually <500 U/L and ALT is <200 U/L. There may be more of a cholestatic disease picture with high AP and GGT levels.

In viral hepatitis, AST and ALT are predominantly elevated. They are in the range of several thousand units per liter in acute hepatic infection. They are generally only 2–3 times normal values if chronic hepatitis is the reason for enzyme elevation.

Markers for viral hepatitis should be tested to screen for viral hepatitis infection and immunity (Hepatitis A and C antibodies, Hepatitis B surface antigen, surface antibody, and core antibody).

In nonalcoholic fatty liver disease, AST and ALT are mildly elevated. A liver ultrasound can be done to look for fatty infiltration of the liver.

> *AST and ALT are more likely to be elevated than other liver enzymes with injury from psychotropic medications; rise in AP, GGT can occur but are more likely to be from other etiologies.*

Management

It is not necessary to measure liver enzymes before initiating every psychotropic medication. However, in the absence of any prior lab data, LFT measurement is useful to obtain a baseline value. There is no need to routinely monitor LFTs while on psychotropic treatment except for valproate and carbamazepine. With all other medications, LFTs should be checked only if any clinical symptoms arise (including nonspecific symptoms like fatigue). If LFTs are done and do show hepatic inflammation, medication can be continued with mild transaminase elevations. Patients can be continued on the offending medication until the transaminases are approximately three times the normal value. The same threshold can be used for carbamazepine and valproate. If the enzymes rise beyond three times normal, it is recommended to stop the medication. Reducing the dose may be attempted but there is no evidence that it will lessen the hepatic inflammation. Rechallenge with the same medication will likely cause recurrence of LFT elevation.

There is no need to routinely check ammonia levels on valproate. If a patient develops clinical signs of hepatic encephalopathy such as gait problems and altered mental status and hyperammonemia is identified, valproate should be stopped. Levocarnitine can be administered to hasten resolution of the hyperammonemia. There is no good evidence on using levocarnitine for prevention of hyperammonemia and maintenance on valproate long term; however, it can be attempted in patients after an episode of hyperammonemia if valproate is clinically necessary. Dose reduction of valproate should be tried first, if possible. All the same strategies can be used for carbamazepine also though there is less evidence to guide recommendations.

> *It is not necessary to routinely monitor LFTs for medications other than valproate and carbamazepine.*
>
> *Transaminase elevation more than three times normal is an indication to stop the offending medication.*
>
> *There is no need to measure ammonia in asymptomatic patients on valproate.*

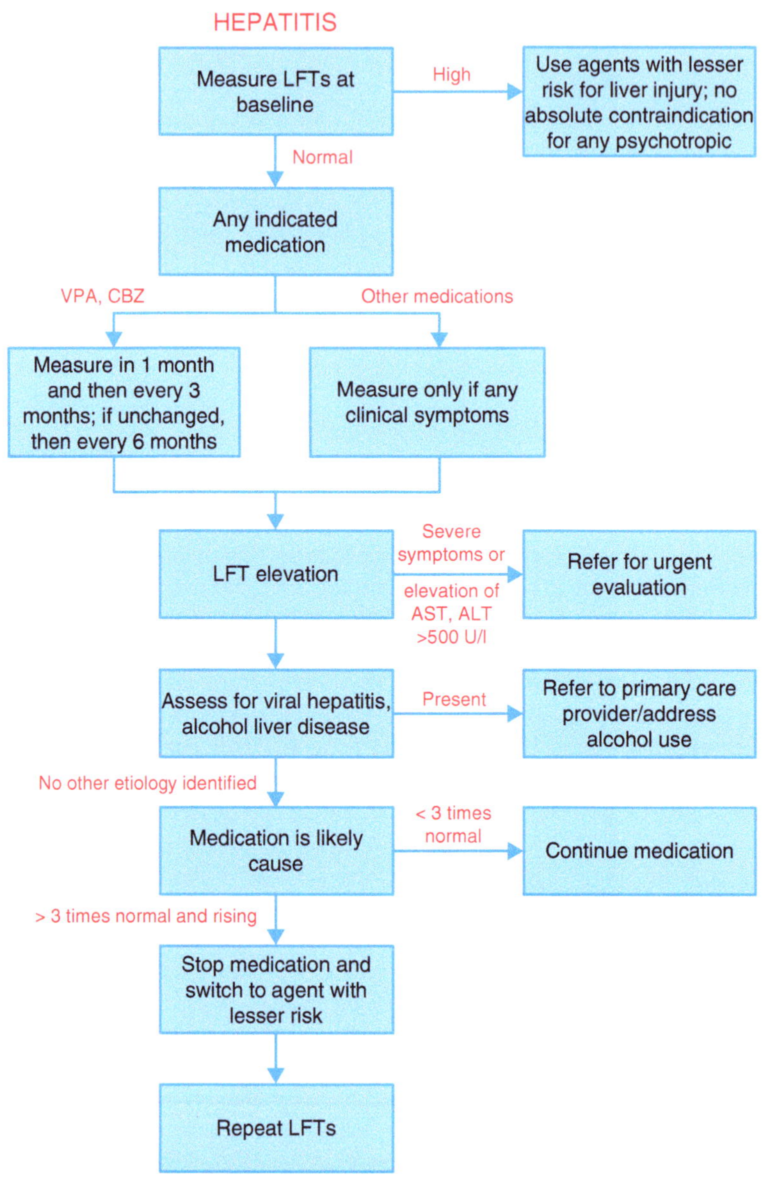

HEPATITIS
Measure LFTs at baseline
High
Use agents with lesser risk for liver injury; no absolute contraindication for any psychotropic
Normal
Any indicated medication
VPA, CBZ
Other medications
Measure in 1 month and then every 3 months; if unchanged, then every 6 months
Measure only if any clinical symptoms
LFT elevation
Severe symptoms or elevation of AST, ALT >500 U/l
Refer for urgent evaluation
Assess for viral hepatitis, alcohol liver disease
Present
Refer to primary care provider/address alcohol use
No other etiology identified
Medication is likely cause
< 3 times normal
Continue medication
> 3 times normal and rising
Stop medication and switch to agent with lesser risk
Repeat LFTs

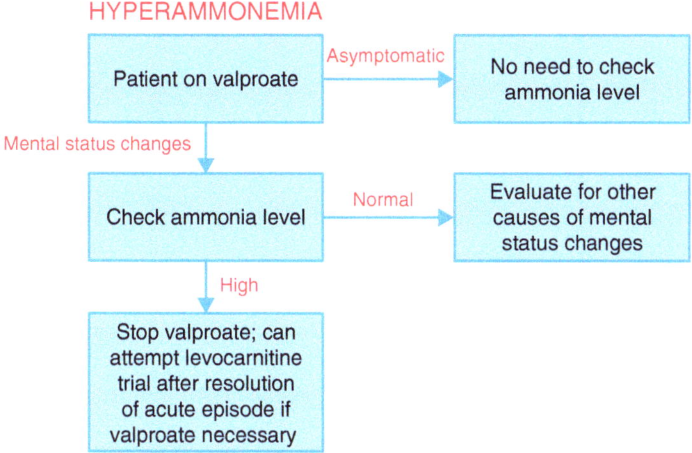

References

1. Marwick KF, Taylor M, Walker SW. Antipsychotics and abnormal liver function tests: systematic review. Clin Neuropharmacol. 2012;35(5):244–53.
2. Atasoy N, Erdogan A, Yalug I, Ozturk U, Konuk N, Atik L, et al. A review of liver function tests during treatment with atypical antipsychotic drugs: a chart review study. Prog Neuropsychopharmacol Biol Psychiatry. 2007;31(6):1255–60.
3. Voican CS, Corruble E, Naveau S, Perlemuter G. Antidepressant-induced liver injury: a review for clinicians. Am J Psychiatry. 2014;171(4):404–15.
4. National Institutes of Health. LiverTox: clinical and research information on drug-induced liver injury. https://livertox.nlm.nih.gov. Accessed 14 Oct 2016.
5. Wadzinski J, Franks R, Roane D, Bayard M. Valproate-associated hyperammonemic encephalopathy. J Am Board Fam Med. 2007;20(5):499–502.
6. Powell-Jackson PR, Tredger JM, Williams R. Hepatotoxicity to sodium valproate: a review. Gut. 1984;25(6).673–81.

Chapter 21
Pancreatitis

Acute pancreatitis is a clinical condition characterized by elevated pancreatic enzymes and abdominal symptoms. It is uncommon but potentially fatal and thus is a leading cause of hospitalization. Chronic pancreatitis can result from repeat episodes of acute pancreatitis.

Pathology

The pathogenesis depends on the particular etiology. Pathogenesis of drug-induced pancreatitis is not well understood.

Etiology

In the United States, gall stones and alcohol use account for the majority of cases of acute pancreatitis. Other less common causes are hypertriglyceridemia, pancreatic duct obstruction, iatrogenic (after cholangiopancreatography), systemic infections, ischemia, and blunt trauma. Medications are a rare cause of pancreatitis; however, many medications, including several psychotropics, are reported to be associated with pancreatitis. Most patients who develop pancreatitis carry multiple risk factors.

© Springer International Publishing AG 2017

A. Annamalai, *Medical Management of Psychotropic Side Effects*,
DOI 10.1007/978-3-319-51026-2_21

Psychotropic Medications and Pancreatitis

It is a rare (<1%) and idiosyncratic phenomenon and is based mostly on case reports. It is reported with valproate, which carries a black box warning regarding its association with pancreatitis. It is less commonly reported with carbamazepine. It is also associated with some antipsychotic medications. Antidepressants do not carry an increased risk for pancreatitis [1].

The exact mechanism of pancreatitis is unknown but two hypotheses are cell damage from toxic free radicals and immunologic reactions.

The pancreatic damage can occur at any time in treatment, though the majority of cases are within 12 months for valproate [2] and within 6 months for antipsychotics [3]. Among antipsychotics, case reports are most frequent with clozapine and olanzapine. In one review of FDA surveillance data and case reports, atypical antipsychotics were more likely to be associated with pancreatitis than haloperidol, which was used as the comparator drug [3]. Among the three atypical antipsychotics reviewed, frequency of association was clozapine > olanzapine > risperidone.

> *Valproate is associated with pancreatitis; among antipsychotics, clozapine and olanzapine are most frequently associated with pancreatitis; incidence with all these agents is low.*

There is no clear correlation between dose of medication and the risk of pancreatitis [2, 3]. Risk factors for pancreatitis are additive. Patients with gallstones, obesity, and elevated triglycerides are at higher risk for developing pancreatitis on these medications.

Clinical Features

Common presenting symptoms are nausea, vomiting, and abdominal pain. In severe cases, fever and hypotension may be present at onset of illness.

> *Acute abdominal pain of unknown origin in a patient started on an offending medication within the last year is a concern for pancreatitis.*

Diagnosis

Serum elevation of pancreatic enzymes, usually three times higher than normal, supports the diagnosis. Lipase rises earlier, stays elevated later, and is more specific than amylase for pancreatic damage. Liver function tests should also be checked to rule out other etiologies. If further confirmation is needed, patients may get an ultrasound or CT or MRI, which are more sensitive. MRCP or ERCP is usually reserved for chronic pancreatitis.

There are no distinguishing features of medication-induced pancreatitis that are different from pancreatitis of any other cause. Serum amylase is sometimes transiently elevated with valproate in the absence of pancreatitis.

Lipase is more specific than amylase for diagnosing pancreatitis.

Management

There is no need to routinely measure serum amylase or lipase during treatment with valproate or antipsychotics. If patients report abdominal pain, nausea, or vomiting, especially when on valproate, clozapine, or olanzapine, lipase and amylase should be measured. If pancreatitis is suspected or confirmed, medication should be stopped. Generally, the combination of symptoms and enzyme elevation is sufficient but imaging can be done if diagnosis is in doubt. Rechallenge is not recommended as in the majority of patients, pancreatitis recurs.

There is no need to routinely measure lipase or amylase during treatment with medications at risk for pancreatitis.

After an episode of medication-induced pancreatitis rechallenge is not recommended with same medication.

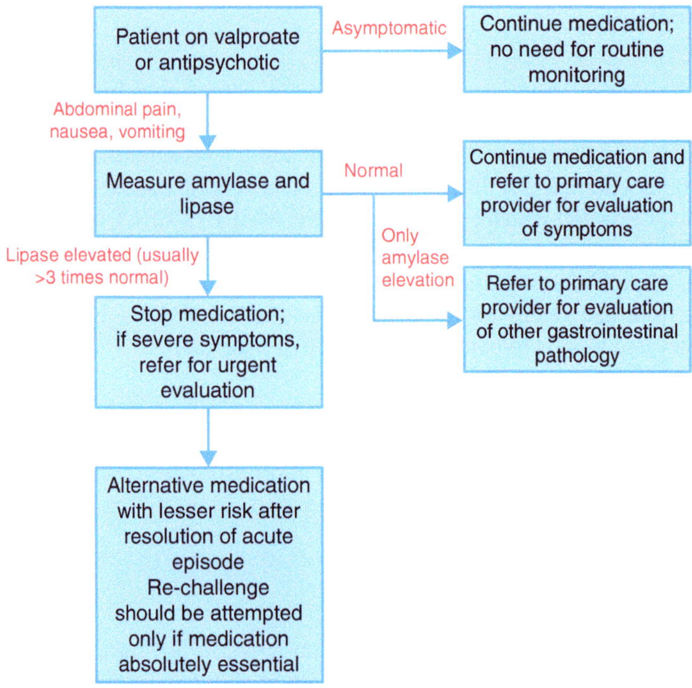

References

1. Ljung R, Ruck C, Mattsson F, Bexelius TS, Lagergren J, Lindblad M. Selective serotonin reuptake inhibitors and the risk of acute pancreatitis: a Swedish population-based case-control study. J Clin Psychopharmacol. 2012;32(3):336–40.
2. Chapman SA, Wacksman GP, Patterson BD. Pancreatitis associated with valproic acid: a review of the literature. Pharmacotherapy. 2001;21(12):1549–60.
3. Koller EA, Cross JT, Doraiswamy PM, Malozowski SN. Pancreatitis associated with atypical antipsychotics: from the Food and Drug Administration's MedWatch surveillance system and published reports. Pharmacotherapy. 2003;23(9):1123–30.

Chapter 22
Constipation

Constipation is traditionally defined as defecation less than three times weekly. But it can also be disruption in bowel movements due to increased straining, sense of incomplete evacuation, or feeling of blockage during defecation. Chronic constipation is reported in at least 15% the general population and up to 57.7% in people with mental illness [1].

Pathology

Colonic motility is coordinated by the autonomic nervous system. Constipation is usually due to slow colonic transit of stool rather than outlet obstruction. Often the colonic slowing is idiopathic and associated with poor dietary habits and psychological issues. Occasionally constipation is due to secondary causes.

Etiology

Systemic illnesses such as diabetes or hypothyroidism can cause constipation. Inflammatory bowel disease can cause constipation though diarrhea is usually more common. Irritable bowel syndrome is usually associated with alternating diarrhea though often, constipation is predominant. Colonic obstruction due to malignancy is also a potential etiology. Constipation is also a side effect of many medications. A notable example among nonpsychotropic medications is opiates. Often, there is no identified etiology.

© Springer International Publishing AG 2017
A. Annamalai, *Medical Management of Psychotropic Side Effects*,
DOI 10.1007/978-3-319-51026-2_22

Psychotropic Medications and Constipation

Constipation is a common side effect of antipsychotics and requires some pharmacological management in at least one-third of patients [2]. The mechanism is mainly via anticholinergic activity. Clozapine is associated with more cases of constipation than other antipsychotics. There are case reports of fatal complications including paralytic ileus, fecal impaction, bowel obstruction, and intestinal perforation [3]. Among other antipsychotics, olanzapine is a frequent cause of constipation. Even haloperidol, a typical antipsychotic, is associated with constipation [3].

> *Atypical antipsychotics and risk for constipation*
>
> *Clozapine > olanzapine > risperidone > quetiapine > ziprasidone > aripiprazole*

Among antidepressants, tricyclic antidepressants (TCAs) cause constipation due to their anticholinergic activity. The effect of serotonin on the intestines is not well understood. Selective serotonergic reuptake inhibitors (SSRIs) are thought to be prokinetic but they have been associated with constipation [1]. Similarly, benzodiazepines may have some effect on colonic motility but the clinical significance is unclear. Antihistamines with anticholinergic activity (e.g., diphenhydramine) also can cause constipation if used regularly. Mood stabilizers are not known to cause constipation.

Constipation resulting from medications resolves quickly if the medication is stopped. Dose reduction can be tried before stopping the medication.

> *Constipation is a common side effect of antipsychotics, especially clozapine; complications of severe constipation can be fatal.*

Clinical Features

Constipation from medications does not have any distinguishing features. Patients may complain of reduced frequency, straining at bowel movements, or blocked feeling during defecation. If constipation is severe, bloating, abdominal pain, and obstipation (a complete lack of passage of stools or flatus) occur. Rarely, in severe cases, there may be changes in appetite or nausea. Abdominal pain with obstipation should also raise suspicion for bowel obstruction. Any systemic signs including change in vital signs should raise suspicion for bowel perforation.

> *Accompanying symptoms of constipation like abdominal pain, lack of flatus, vomiting, should raise suspicion for serious complications of constipation.*

Diagnosis

Generally, no testing is needed for evaluation of constipation. Plain radiography is useful to look for stool retention and complications of constipation. If constipation is accompanied by red flags for colonic malignancy (e.g., blood in stools, weight loss), endoscopic testing is warranted. Patients with refractory constipation may need to be referred for advanced testing such as colonic transit studies or anorectal manometry.

> ***Testing is necessary only if diagnosis of constipation is uncertain, complications are suspected, or other medical illnesses need to be ruled out.***

Management

Chronic constipation should be attributed to medications if no other known etiologies are present and the onset of symptom corresponds to medication initiation. If it does not, common conditions such as hypothyroidism and serious conditions like malignancy should be ruled out.

Management is a combination of patient education, dietary changes, and pharmacologic therapy. Patients should be educated on normality of bowel movements and what is considered healthy frequency, importance of timing bowel movements in the morning and after meals (times of peak colonic activity), and need for maintaining adequate fiber and fluids in diet.

Pharmacologic agents should be tried in the order listed in the table below. A stepped-up treatment approach is also shown for managing inadequate response. Bulk-forming laxatives are the most physiologic treatments. Combinations of agents from two different classes may be tried if suboptimal improvement with one type of agent. If possible, stimulant laxatives should be avoided on a routine basis. In cases of fecal impaction, enemas may be necessary.

The decision to continue the potentially offending medication depends on the severity of constipation. Dose reduction can also be tried. Generally, constipation responds to increasing intensity of pharmacologic therapy and treatment needs to be continued long term.

At any stage of treatment, if constipation is severe and accompanied by other symptoms like abdominal pain or fever, patients should be referred for emergent evaluation to rule out bowel obstruction and other serious complications.

If constipation is resistant to treatment or complications such as bowel obstruction and ileus occur, medication should be stopped and not restarted. Clozapine may be an exception as it cannot easily be substituted. There are occasional case reports of successful use of bethanechol, a cholinomimetic agent, to treat clozapine-induced refractory constipation [4].

Agents to treat constipation

Agent class	Mechanism	Dosing	Side effects
Bulk-forming laxatives			
Psyllium (Metamucil)	Increase water secretion in bowel and increase bulk	One spoon three times daily, can increase up to two spoons	Abdominal fullness and bloating
Wheat dextrin (Benefiber)			
Methylcellulose			
Prunes			
Stool softeners			
Docusate sodium	Lower surface tension of stool	100 mg twice daily, can go up to 200 mg twice daily	Well tolerated
Osmotic agents			
Polyethylene glycol	Increase intestinal water secretion and stool frequency	8–34 g in 8 oz. liquid	Abdominal bloating, flatulence, watery stools with urgency
Lactulose		15–30 mL every other day to daily	
Magnesium citrate		200 mL daily	
Stimulant laxatives			
Bisacodyl	Increase intestinal motility	10–30 mg daily	Urgency, diarrhea
Senna (use in suppository form if fecal impaction)		Up to four tablets once or twice daily	
Others			
Linaclotide	Stimulates intestinal fluid secretion and transit	145 µg daily	Diarrhea
Lubiprostone	Increases intestinal fluid secretion	24 µg twice daily	Diarrhea, bloating

Stepped-up treatment approach

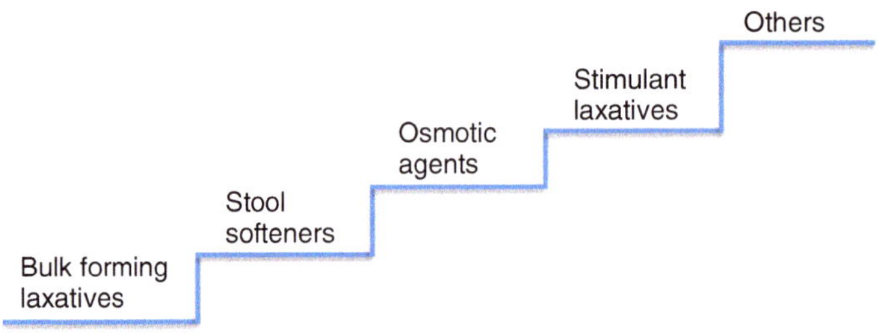

Dietary modifications and stepped-up pharmacological approach will treat most cases of medication-induced constipation.

When serious complications result from psychotropic-induced constipation, medication should preferably be stopped; clozapine may be an exception.

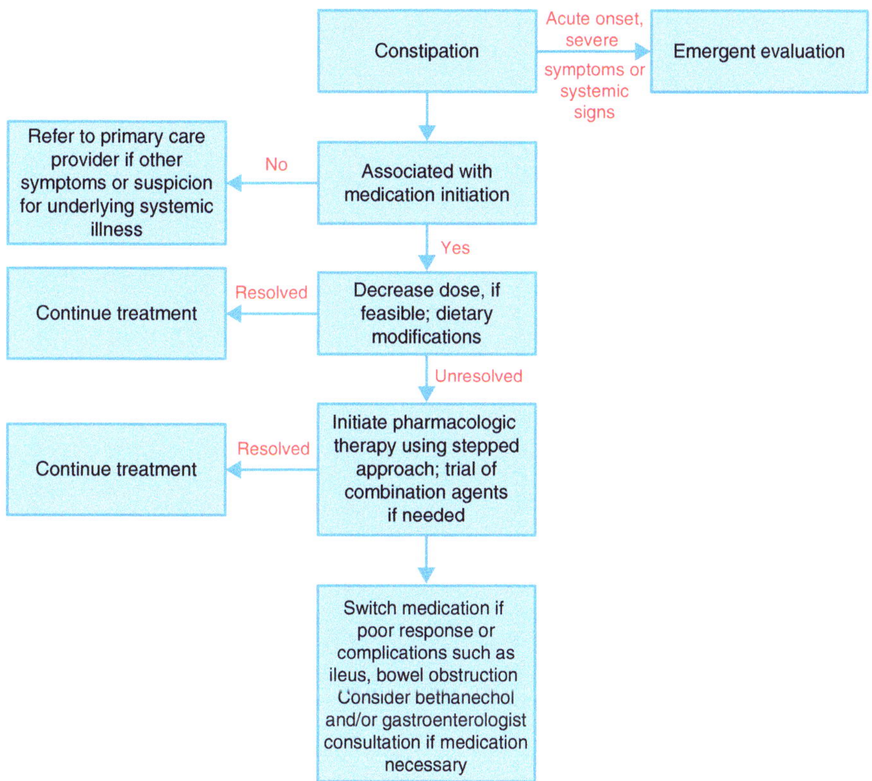

References

1. Jessurun JG, van Harten PN, Egberts TC, Pijl BJ, Wilting I, Tenback DE. The effect of psychotropic medications on the occurrence of constipation in hospitalized psychiatric patients. J Clin Psychopharmacol. 2013;33(4):587–90.
2. De Hert M, Dockx L, Bernagie C, Peuskens B, Sweers K, Leucht S, et al. Prevalence and severity of antipsychotic related constipation in patients with schizophrenia: a retrospective descriptive study. BMC Gastroenterol. 2011;11:17.
3. De Hert M, Hudyana H, Dockx L, Bernagie C, Sweers K, Tack J, et al. Second-generation antipsychotics and constipation: a review of the literature. Eur Psychiatry. 2011;26(1):34–44.
4. Poetter CE, Stewart JT. Treatment of clozapine-induced constipation with bethanechol. J Clin Psychopharmacol. 2013;33(5):713–4.

Chapter 23
Sialorrhea

Sialorrhea refers to excessive oral secretions causing drooling.

Pathology

It is most commonly due to impaired swallowing due to autonomic dysfunction. Some medications cause sialorrhea by their effects on the cholinergic system.

Etiology

Any neurodegenerative disease with autonomic dysfunction (e.g., Parkinson disease) can cause sialorrhea. Severe impairment in swallowing due to upper gastrointestinal disorders can cause sialorrhea. Among medications, antipsychotics and cholinergic agonists used in Alzheimer's dementia are the usual offenders.

Psychotropic Medications and Sialorrhea

Clozapine is the most likely agent to cause significant sialorrhea though other antipsychotics can increase salivation to a small degree. Even though clozapine has significant anticholinergic properties, it increases salivation by cholinergic agonism. The effect is thought to result from an imbalance between agonism and antagonism between different muscarinic receptors in salivary gland tissue. It may also be related to its alpha adrenergic antagonistic properties, which leads to unopposed beta adrenergic stimulation.

© Springer International Publishing AG 2017

A. Annamalai, *Medical Management of Psychotropic Side Effects*,
DOI 10.1007/978-3-319-51026-2_23

Sialorrhea occurs in 30–80% of patients on clozapine [1]. It occurs early in treatment and is usually more copious at night. Reduction of dose does not reliably improve the symptom.

In addition to the obvious inconvenience, untreated sialorrhea can cause mouth irritation and salivary gland enlargement.

Nonpharmacological treatments have only shown minimal evidence in reducing the sialorrhea. Pharmacological agents with some efficacy are glycopyrrolate, an anticholinergic agent, and terazosin, a peripheral alpha adrenergic blocker [1]. Other anticholinergic agents with some efficacy are benztropine and trihexyphenidyl. Clonidine and guanfacine are central alpha agonists that have shown some efficacy. Other options are sublingual atropine and ipratropium bromide. Botulinum toxin may relieve symptoms but is not well studied [1].

> ***Sialorrhea is a common side effect of clozapine.***

Clinical Features

Patients complain of drooling predominantly during sleep but when it is severe, it occurs during the day also. If there are copious salivary secretions during sleep, there is a risk of laryngeal aspiration.

> ***Clozapine-induced sialorrhea is more prominent during sleep.***

Diagnosis

Sialorrhea is a clinical diagnosis. If autonomic or gastrointestinal disorders are suspected, further diagnostic testing should confirm or rule out those conditions.

> ***Diagnosis of clozapine-induced sialorrhea is easily made unless other etiologies like neurologic or gastrointestinal disorders are present.***

Management

If the sialorrhea is mild and patient is able to manage the symptom, no additional medication is needed. Chewing sugarless gum may help by increasing swallowing. If the drooling is predominantly at night, using a towel over the pillow may be sufficient to contain it.

If drooling is disabling for the patient, dose reduction can be attempted if clinically feasible. With persistent drooling, an anticholinergic may be considered. Glycopyrrolate is a good first choice but benztropine and trihexyphenidyl are also reasonable options. If patient already has other anticholinergic side effects from clozapine, terazosin, an alpha antagonist, may be used as a first-line agent. Combination of terazosin and an anticholinergic medication may work better than either agent alone. If none of these strategies are effective, clonidine and guanfacine, both alpha agonists, can be tried. Sublingual atropine is reserved for refractory sialorrhea in patients who need to continue clozapine.

Many pharmacologic therapies exist for clozapine-induced sialorrhea but often symptom does not resolve completely.

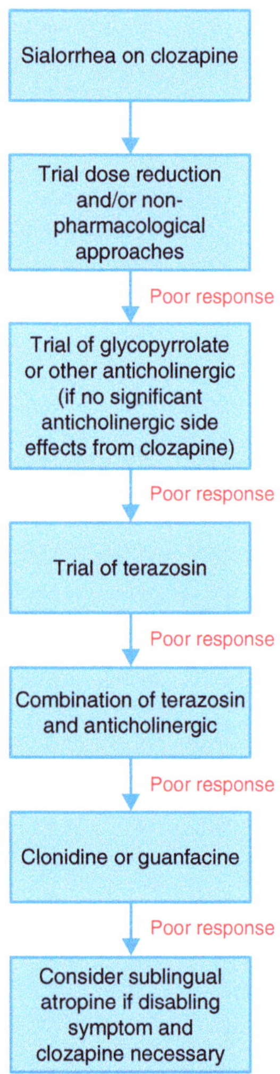

Reference

1. Bird AM, Smith TL, Walton AE. Current treatment strategies for clozapine-induced sialorrhea. Ann Pharmacother. 2011;45(5):667–75.

Chapter 24
Bruxism

Bruxism is involuntary clenching and grinding of teeth. It often occurs during sleep but can be present during the day also.

Pathology

People with bruxism may have a genetic predisposition. An imbalance in central dopaminergic neurotransmission is hypothesized to play a role.

Etiology

Bruxism is associated with oral problems like temporomandibular joint dysfunction (TMJ), psychological distress, sleep disorders, increased esophageal acidity, and some psychotropic medications.

Psychotropic Medications and Bruxism

Psychotropic medications may cause bruxism by affecting motor activity by direct effect on dopaminergic pathways or indirectly via serotonergic pathways. The side effect may occur on starting treatment or increasing dosage.

Most information on bruxism and psychotropic medications is derived from case reports. Serotonin reuptake inhibitors (SSRIs), serotonin norepinephrine reuptake (SNRIs), and typical antipsychotics are associated with bruxism [1]. Bruxism with typical antipsychotics seems to occur along with other extrapyramidal symptoms. Stimulants and antihistamines are also known to cause bruxism.

© Springer International Publishing AG 2017

A. Annamalai, *Medical Management of Psychotropic Side Effects*,

DOI 10.1007/978-3-319-51026-2_24

Buspirone is reported to alleviate SSRI-induced bruxism. Some atypical antipsychotics may be successful in treating bruxism and there are case reports with clozapine and aripiprazole. Propranolol and clonidine have been studied to treat bruxism but evidence is limited.

> **Bruxism is infrequently associated with psychotropic medications; among these agents, SSRIs are more likely to be implicated.**

Clinical Features

Patients with bruxism complain of grinding and clenching of teeth. It occurs more commonly during sleep but can occur during the day also. When it is limited to sleep, patient is less aware than family members. Medications can induce bruxism either when awake or during sleep. SSRIs are more likely to cause sleep bruxism.

> **Bruxism due to medications can occur when awake or during sleep.**

Diagnosis

The diagnosis is clinical. Other testing may be needed to rule out coexisting sleep disorders. A dental evaluation may be required if the symptom is either severe or long standing, and dental erosions are suspected.

> **Sleep disorders should be ruled out with bruxism; a dental evaluation is prudent to assess for both causes and complications of bruxism.**

Management

Other etiologies like sleep disorders and TMJ should be ruled out especially if the onset of bruxism is not clearly correlated with starting medications. If patient has mild bruxism on SSRI treatment, no intervention may be needed. However, ongoing dental evaluation is recommended to assess and monitor dental health. Occasionally, bruxism may resolve spontaneously. If there are persistent impairing symptoms, buspirone can be tried. If associated with anxiety, benzodiazepines may help. Wearing a dental guard may help in cases of persistent nocturnal bruxism.

There is no evidence on differential risk of bruxism between different SSRIs or between SSRIs and SNRIs. Tricyclic antidepressants are an option if bruxism occurs with different SSRIs and SNRIs and does not respond to treatment.

If the bruxism is associated with typical antipsychotics, switching to an atypical agent, especially clozapine and aripiprazole may be reasonable options in the appropriate clinical situation. Propranolol can be tried if there are also extrapyramidal symptoms of akathisia.

Bruxism should be treated if symptoms are impairing or there is risk of dental erosions.

Buspirone is first-line treatment for SSRI-induced bruxism.

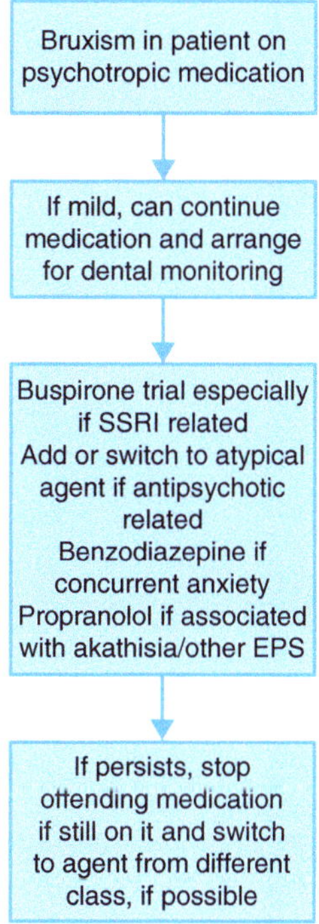

Reference

1. Falisi G, Rastelli C, Panti F, Maglione H, Quezada Arcega R. Psychotropic drugs and bruxism. Expert Opin Drug Saf. 2014;13(10):1319–26.

Section VIII
Hematologic System

Chapter 25
Introduction to Blood Cell Disorders

Many drugs besides psychotropic medications are associated with hematologic abnormalities. One or more cell lines may be affected depending on the drug and its mechanism of action. Drug-induced blood dyscrasias occur infrequently other than when associated with chemotherapy. The exact incidence varies with each medication.

Pathology

The two basic mechanisms are suppression of hematopoiesis by direct toxicity to the bone marrow and formation of antibodies against blood cells.

Drug Etiologies

Major nonpsychotropic medications associated with blood dyscrasias are listed in the following table. Patients on psychotropic treatment are also likely to be on many of these other agents and it is important to evaluate for synergistic effects from different medications.

Nonpsychotropic medications associated with blood dyscrasias
Several antibiotics
Anticonvulsants
Nonsteroidal anti-inflammatory drugs
Antihypertensives
Cardiac agents
Sulfonylureas
Antifungals
Antimalarial drugs

© Springer International Publishing AG 2017

A. Annamalai, *Medical Management of Psychotropic Side Effects*,
DOI 10.1007/978-3-319-51026-2_25

Psychotropic Medications and Blood Dyscrasias

As with other medications, psychotropic drug-induced blood dyscrasias are infrequent. Among them, drug-induced neutropenia is the most frequent but even this side effect is <1% [1]. Mechanism of dyscrasia is either suppression of hematopoiesis or immune-mediated destruction of one or more blood cell lines.

Many psychotropic medications cause a mild degree of blood dyscrasia. The following table lists psychotropic agents commonly associated with blood dyscrasias as well as agents rarely associated with dyscrasias. Each dyscrasia induced by psychotropic agents is discussed separately in the following chapters.

Blood dyscrasias and associated psychotropic medications [2]

Type of dyscrasia	Common associations	Rare association (often only case reports)
Agranulocytosis	Clozapine, carbamazepine, mirtazapine, phenothiazine antipsychotics	Tricyclic antidepressants (TCAs) (in combination with other agents), atypical antipsychotics
Leukopenia	Same agents as above, valproate, lamotrigine	Atypical antipsychotics, Selective Serotonin Reuptake Inhibitors (SSRIs), venlafaxine, bupropion, benzodiazepines
Leukocytosis	Lithium	–
Thrombocytopenia	Mirtazapine, carbamazepine, valproate, lamotrigine	TCAs, phenothiazine antipsychotics
	SSRIs cause impaired platelet aggregation	
Anemia	Carbamazepine, mirtazapine, lamotrigine	Venlafaxine, sertraline, citalopram, benzodiazepines
Eosinophilia	Carbamazepine, lamotrigine	Olanzapine, TCAs, valproate

References

1. Stubner S, Grohmann R, Engel R, Bandelow B, Ludwig WD, Wagner G, et al. Blood dyscrasias induced by psychotropic drugs. Pharmacopsychiatry. 2004;37(Suppl 1):S70–8.
2. Oyesanmi O, Kunkel EJ, Monti DA, Field HL. Hematologic side effects of psychotropics. Psychosomatics. 1999;40(5):414–21.

Chapter 26
Leukopenia

Leukopenia is an abnormally low number of circulating leukocytes or white blood cells. The cutoff for normal leukocyte count varies between labs but usually ranges between 3500 and 4000 cells/µL.

It is the most common hematologic abnormality seen with psychotropic medications. The majority of drug-induced reductions in leukocytes cause neutropenia, a reduction in neutrophils.

Neutropenia is usually defined as an absolute neutrophil count (ANC) <1500 cells/µL. ANC is the product of the white blood cell (WBC) count and the percentage of neutrophils and is reported along with the automated cell counts in almost all laboratories.

Neutropenia is classified according to severity as shown in the table.

Classification of neutropenia

Neutropenia	ANC (cells/µL)
Mild	>1000<1500
Moderate	>500<1000
Severe	<500

Agranulocytosis is defined as the complete absence of circulating neutrophils but is sometimes applied to profound neutropenia with ANC < 500.

Pathology

Neutrophils are produced by myeloid precursor cells in the bone marrow and migrate to the circulation and other tissues. In addition to decreased production and increased destruction, shift of neutrophils from circulation to tissues can result in a reduced neutrophil count.

© Springer International Publishing AG 2017
A. Annamalai, *Medical Management of Psychotropic Side Effects,*
DOI 10.1007/978-3-319-51026-2_26

Etiology

Major causes of neutropenia are benign ethic neutropenia and drug-induced states. The following table lists these and other causes of neutropenia.

Causes of neutropenia

Benign chronic (blacks, certain Arab, Jewish and West Indian groups)
Drug induced (commonly chemotherapy; also antibiotics and psychotropics)
Postinfectious (bacterial, viral, or parasitic)
Immune mediated (collagen vascular disorders)
Nutritional deficiencies (commonly folate, Vitamin B12)
Bone marrow disorders (Myelodysplasia)
Congenital neutropenia syndromes (usually diagnosed in childhood); Cyclic neutropenia is one type but usually benign

Benign ethnic neutropenia

Prevalence: As high as 10%; more common in African descent
Degree: Usually ANC>1000<1500
Mechanism: Not clearly understood. Generally these people have a preserved bone marrow neutrophil reserve and are not at increased risk of infections
Clinical presentation: Often encountered when performing lab tests for routine screening. It may be detected for the first time in a psychiatric setting
Diagnosis: Based on history and chronic low ANC with no other identified etiology
Management: Generally, these people do not need referral to a hematologist as long as the ANC remains stable. There is no threshold for referral for a bone marrow evaluation but may be considered if ANC < 1000 or it trends down

Psychotropic Medications and Neutropenia

Almost all major classes of psychotropic medications have been associated with neutropenia. The mechanism of drug-induced neutropenia is either decreased production in bone marrow due to direct toxic effect or sensitization of neutrophils to peripheral destruction. The effect is usually seen within 1–2 weeks of treatment. Withdrawing medication usually leads to resolution in 3–4 weeks [1].

Agranulocytosis is a rare side effect but is associated with up to 10% mortality when it occurs. It occurs later in treatment, about 3–4 weeks after exposure, and also resolves within 3–4 weeks of stopping the medication [1].

When the mechanism is bone marrow suppression, drug-induced neutropenia may be dose related and predictable whereas when the mechanism is immune-mediated destruction, it is idiosyncratic. However, with most medications, the mechanism is not clearly defined and they may both suppress bone marrow production and initiate peripheral destruction. Agranulocytosis is thought to be more commonly an idiosyncratic reaction unrelated to dose. But neutropenia can be a precursor for the more serious agranulocytosis. Unfortunately, there is no reliable way to predict which patients with neutropenia will progress to agranulocytosis. Agranulocytosis may also occur without antecedent neutropenia. Risk for neutropenia is higher at younger ages while risk for agranulocytosis is higher in the elderly.

> ***Mechanism of psychotropic-induced neutropenia is either dose-related bone marrow suppression or idiosyncratic peripheral destruction.***
>
> ***Neutropenia usually occurs within 1–2 weeks and agranulocytosis within 3–4 weeks; both resolve in 3–4 weeks of stopping medication.***
>
> ***There is no reliable way to predict which cases of neutropenia will progress to agranulocytosis.***

Among the offending psychotropic agents, incidence is highest with unmonitored use of clozapine. Risk of neutropenia is 3% and agranulocytosis is 0.7–1%. Chlorpromazine and olanzapine are two other antipsychotics that have a high incidence of neutropenia [1]. Most antipsychotics are also associated with agranulocytosis.

Mood stabilizers are associated with neutropenia [2]. Carbamazepine is also associated with agranulocytosis [3].

Among antidepressants, mirtazapine is associated with agranulocytosis. There are case reports of agranulocytosis with tricyclic antidepressants (TCAs). There are also case reports with some benzodiazepines.

Psychotropic medications causing neutropenia

Most likely agents	Clozapine, carbamazepine, phenothiazine antipsychotics
Less likely agents	Valproate, lamotrigine, TCAs, mirtazapine, atypical antipsychotics
Least likely agents	Selective serotonin reuptake inhibitors (SSRIs), venlafaxine, bupropion, benzodiazepines

Rechallenge with the offending medication may need to be considered, especially with clozapine. Rechallenge after previous neutropenia on clozapine results in recurrence in at least a third of patients [4]. It is likely to occur sooner, be more severe, and last longer. The reason may be due to previous immune 'priming.' But there is a population of patients in whom rechallenge does not lead to neutropenia. There are case reports of successful clozapine rechallenge even after occurrence of agranulocytosis [4].

Lithium raises leukocyte count and is used during clozapine rechallenge to counter the neutrophil suppression. However, it does not prevent agranulocytosis, which may occur due to a different mechanism. Hence, it may mask the development of agranulocytosis when it is used with clozapine. Granulocyte colony-stimulating factor (G-CSF) has also been used to prevent neutropenia with clozapine rechallenge.

> *Clozapine rechallenge results in recurrent neutropenia in about a third of patients; when it does occur, it is likely to be more severe.*

Clinical Features

Mild to moderate neutropenia is generally asymptomatic. Severe neutropenia increases the risk of systemic infections. Initial symptoms may be oral ulcers and fever. Drug-induced severe neutropenia may present with sudden onset of headache, fever, and malaise.

> *Though fever may not always be a presenting symptom in severe neutropenia, its presence should warrant immediate testing of neutrophil count in patients on potentially offending medications.*

Diagnosis

An ANC <1500 cells/μL is a diagnosis of neutropenia. If available, prior records are important for determining if the neutropenia is acute or chronic. The test should be repeated to rule out an acute postinfectious state.

ANC should be repeated at the same time of day if feasible, as there can be some diurnal variation. Exercise and cigarette smoking just prior to lab draw can also alter ANC.

Vitamin B12 and folate levels, hepatitis, HIV should be tested to rule out nutritional deficiencies and chronic infections. Further evaluations of neutropenia such as bone marrow aspiration are only needed if neutropenia is severe and sustained.

> *Other etiologies should be ruled out by lab testing before ascribing neutropenia to medications; neutrophil count should be tested at the same time of day, if possible.*

Management

For medications at high risk for causing neutropenia, ANC should be measured before initiating medication. No clear guidelines exist except for clozapine. But baseline testing and continued monitoring should be done for carbamazepine. It can be considered for other antipsychotics.

When neutropenia is detected, other causes such as infections or nutritional deficiencies should be ruled out. As mentioned earlier, ANC should preferably be measured at a similar time of day each time and factors such as exercise and smoking immediately preceding lab testing should be considered. If the neutropenia is severe and patient is on a high-risk medication, it should be stopped while the cause is being evaluated.

When neutropenia persists and is suspected to be from the psychotropic agent, medication can be continued if neutropenia is mild. The medication should be stopped if neutropenia is moderate to severe or there is a progressive decline. If the medication is stopped, the ANC generally returns to normal within 1–2 weeks.

ANC monitoring on clozapine follows national guidelines in the United States. According to recently revised guidelines, clozapine can be continued without interruption for ANC>1000 cells/μL and in patients with benign ethnic neutropenia for ANC>500 cells/μL. The Risk Evaluation and Mitigation Strategies (REMS) program of Food and Drug Administration (FDA) ensures monitoring risks and benefits for medications. The REMS program for clozapine contains resources for prescribers on ANC monitoring. See appendix for the summary table. More details can be found at the clozapine REMS website (https://www.clozapinerems.com/CpmgClozapineUI/resources.u#tabr4).

Since clozapine is often chosen for lack of effectiveness of other medications, it may not be possible to switch to alternative medications and additional strategies may be necessary to maintain the ANC within acceptable limits.

As mentioned earlier, lithium is used to stimulate neutrophil production. Lithium has been used both to increase ANC before initiating clozapine and for rechallenge after clozapine-induced neutropenia. The magnitude of neutrophil increase with lithium is not consistent. There is no clear dose–effect relationship but generally serum lithium level >0.4 mEq/L. is thought to be necessary. Clinicians should remember that lithium does not protect against agranulocytosis.

G-CSF increases maturation of granulocytes in bone marrow and is used extensively during chemotherapy and in nonpharmacologic causes of neutropenia. Evidence is limited for use in clozapine-induced neutropenia but case reports exist for use of G-CSF to raise ANC both before initiating clozapine and for clozapine rechallenge after neutropenia. Generally, weekly doses are used. G CSF is significantly more expensive than lithium and more difficult to administer as it requires weekly clinic visits and collaboration with hematology.

Rechallenge after agranulocytosis on clozapine is not recommended though there are occasional case reports of successful rechallenge. It can be considered in extenuating circumstances where clozapine is absolutely necessary for psychiatric symptom control. All other potential contributors including other psychotropic agents should be eliminated.

Routine ANC monitoring is necessary only for high-risk medications like clozapine and carbamazepine.

Generally, there is no need to stop medication for mild psychotropic-induced neutropenia; it should be considered for carbamazepine; clozapine prescribing follows standard guidelines.

Medication should be stopped for moderate to severe neutropenia.

Rechallenge with clozapine after occurrence of neutropenia can be considered with concurrent lithium or G-CSF.

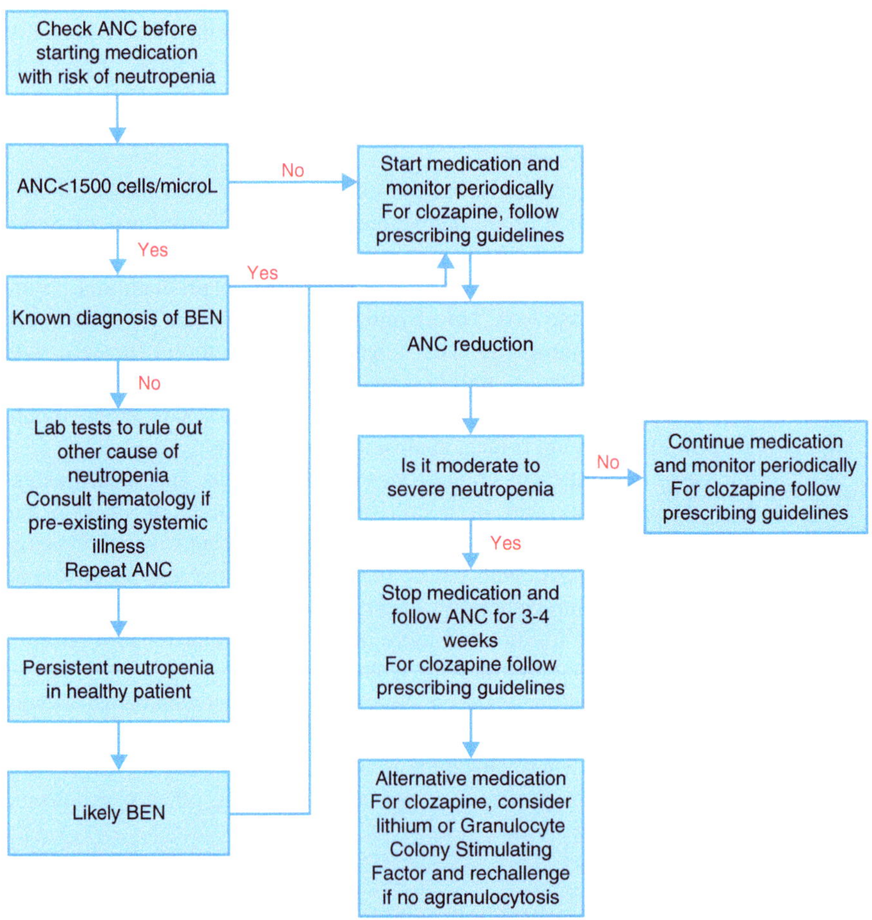

Appendix

Recommended ANC monitoring on clozapine (REMS)

ANC Level	Treatment Recommendation	ANC Monitoring

Normal Range for a New Patient
GENERAL POPULATION
· ANC ≥ 1500/µL
 	
BEN POPULATION
· ANC ≥ 1000/µL
· Obtain at least two baseline ANC levels before initiating treatment
	· Initiate treatment
	· If treatment interrupted:
	  - < 30 days, continue monitoring as before
	  - ≥ 30 days, monitor as if new patient
	
	· Discontinuation for reasons other than neutropenia
		· Weekly from initiation to six months
		· Every 2 weeks from 6 to 12 months
		· Monthly after 12 months
		
		· See Section 2.4 of the full Prescribing Information

Mild Neutropenia
(1000 - 1499/µL)*
	GENERAL POPULATION
	· Continue treatment
	
	BEN POPULATION
	· Mild Neutropenia is normal range for BEN population, continue treatment
	· Obtain at least two baseline ANC levels before initiating treatment
	· If treatment interrupted
	  - < 30 days, continue monitoring as before
	  - ≥ 30 days, monitor as if new patient
	
	· Discontinuation for reasons other than neutropenia
		GENERAL POPULATION
		· Three times weekly until ANC ≥ 1500/µL
		· Once ANC ≥ 1500/µL return to patient's last "Normal Range" ANC monitoring interval**
		
		BEN POPULATION
		· Weekly from initiation to six months
		· Every 2 weeks from 6 to 12 months
		· Monthly after 12 months
		
		· See Section 2.4 of the full Prescribing Information

Moderate Neutropenia (500 - 999/µL)*	**GENERAL POPULATION** · Recommend hematology consultation · Interrupt treatment for suspected clozapine induced neutropenia · Resume treatment once ANC normalizes to ≥ 1000/µL **BEN POPULATION** · Recommend hematology consultation · Continue treatment	**GENERAL POPULATION** · Daily until ANC ≥ 1000/µL, then · Three times weekly until ANC ≥ 1500/µL · Once ANC ≥ 1500/µL check ANC weekly for 4 weeks, then return to patient's last "Normal Range" ANC monitoring interval** **BEN POPULATION** · Three times weekly until ANC ≥ 1000/µL or ≥ patient's known baseline. · Once ANC ≥ 1000/µL or patient's known baseline, check ANC weekly for 4 weeks, then return to patient's last "Normal BEN Range" ANC monitoring interval.**
Severe Neutropenia (< 500/µL)*	**GENERAL POPULATION** · Recommend hematology consultation · Interrupt treatment for suspected clozapine induced neutropenia · Do not rechallenge unless prescriber determines benefits outweigh risks **BEN POPULATION** · Recommend hematology consultation · Interrupt treatment for suspected clozapine induced neutropenia · Do not rechallenge unless prescriber determines benefits outweigh risks	**GENERAL POPULATION** · Daily until ANC ≥ 1000/µL · Three times weekly until ANC ≥ 1500/µL · If patient rechallenged, resume treatment as a new patient under "Normal Range" monitoring once ANC ≥1500/µL **BEN POPULATION** · Daily until ANC ≥ 500/µL · Three times weekly until ANC ≥ patients established baseline · If patient rechallenged, resume treatment as a new patient under "Normal Range" monitoring once ANC ≥1000/µL or at patient's baseline

* Confirm all initial reports of ANC less than 1500/µL (ANC < 1000/µL for BEN patients) with a repeat ANC measurement within 24 hours
** If clinically appropriate

Courtesy: Clozapine REMS Program (https://www.clozapinerems.com/CpmgClozapineUI/resources.u#tabr4)

References

1. Flanagan RJ, Dunk L. Haematological toxicity of drugs used in psychiatry. Hum Psychopharmacol. 2008;23(Suppl 1):27–41.
2. Stubner S, Grohmann R, Engel R, Bandelow B, Ludwig WD, Wagner G, et al. Blood dyscrasias induced by psychotropic drugs. Pharmacopsychiatry. 2004;37(Suppl 1):S70–8.
3. Oyesanmi O, Kunkel EJ, Monti DA, Field HL. Hematologic side effects of psychotropics. Psychosomatics. 1999;40(5):414–21.
4. Dunk LR, Annan LJ, Andrews CD. Rechallenge with clozapine following leucopenia or neutropenia during previous therapy. Br J Psychiatry. 2006;188:255–63.

Chapter 27
Platelet Function Disorders

Disorders of platelet function include a disruption in platelet function that is independent of actual platelet count.

Pathology

Normal platelet function involves platelet activation, recruitment to site of vascular injury and adhesion, aggregation and accumulation, and platelet binding of coagulation factors. Acquired causes affect one or more of these steps in platelet function.

Etiology

Common etiologies are medications (aspirin, nonsteroidal anti-inflammatory agents), liver, and renal disease.

Psychotropic Medications and Platelet Function Abnormality

Serotonin reuptake inhibitors (SSRIs) block serotonin in platelets and also slightly inhibit platelet aggregation. They are associated with a slightly increased risk of gastrointestinal bleeding, operative blood loss, epistaxis, and cerebral hemorrhage in case reports and epidemiological studies. The absolute risk increase is still very small even with gastrointestinal bleeding, where there is a doubling of risk [1]. The risk is increased in combination with nonsteroidal anti-inflammatory drugs (NSAIDs) and reduced with acid-suppressing medications. There is no clear evidence on differential effect among SSRIs but the SSRIs with high degree of

© Springer International Publishing AG 2017

A. Annamalai, *Medical Management of Psychotropic Side Effects*,

DOI 10.1007/978-3-319-51026-2_27

serotonin reuptake inhibition are more likely to have decreased platelet aggregability. SSRIs may be more likely than Serotonin norepinephrine reuptake inhibitors (SNRIs) to cause gastrointestinal bleeding [2]. Clomipramine, which has significant serotonergic activity, probably carries a risk equivalent to SSRIs.

> ***The absolute risk of bleeding with SSRIs is small; gastrointestinal tract is the most likely source.***

Clinical Features

The clinical manifestation will be similar to that seen with a low platelet count. Initial manifestations may be seen as easy skin bruising or increased mucosal bleeding. Patients may also present with epistaxis, menorrhagia, or intestinal bleeding.

> ***Minor skin bruising or mucosal bleeding may be seen; patients may also directly present with intestinal bleeding.***

Diagnosis

Platelet count can be normal, reduced, or even elevated with functional disorders. Bleeding time is prolonged but not often used as a diagnostic test as it is increased in other hemostatic disorders also. Many tests are now available to test platelet aggregation and other platelet functions. But these are not commonly used in clinical practice to assess medication-induced platelet disorders.

> ***No diagnostic test is useful or necessary to establish SSRI-induced platelet disorder as the cause of abnormal bleeding.***

Management

No monitoring is required routinely in patients on SSRIs. SNRIs may be preferred in patients at higher risk of bleeding due to antiplatelet drugs, chronic liver disease, peptic ulcer disease, or previous history of bleeding. Some SSRIs also inhibit metabolism of warfarin, an anticoagulant, and thus increase risk of bleeding from warfarin.

SSRIs can be used in patients with higher risk of bleeding as long as clinicians are aware and monitor for symptoms of bleeding. If any bleeding is seen after initiating medication, a medication switch should be considered. During treatment with

SSRIs it is preferable to limit NSAID use. Some clinicians recommend concurrently using acid-suppressing medications to reduce gastrointestinal bleeding risk in patients on both SSRIs and NSAIDs. Bleeding time is not useful to differentiate between medication-induced platelet dysfunction and other hemostatic disorders. Platelet aggregation tests are not easily available and not routinely done and in any case they are not specific to SSRI-induced platelet dysfunction.

SSRIs can be used in patients at higher risk of bleeding though SNRIs may be preferable as they carry a lesser risk.

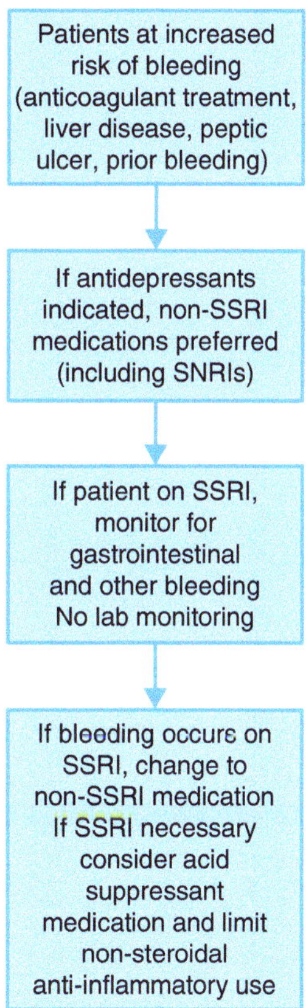

References

1. Andrade C, Sandarsh S, Chethan KB, Nagesh KS. Serotonin reuptake inhibitor antidepressants and abnormal bleeding: a review for clinicians and a reconsideration of mechanisms. J Clin Psychiatry. 2010;71(12):1565–75.
2. de Abajo FJ, Garcia-Rodriguez LA. Risk of upper gastrointestinal tract bleeding associated with selective serotonin reuptake inhibitors and venlafaxine therapy: interaction with nonsteroidal anti-inflammatory drugs and effect of acid-suppressing agents. Arch Gen Psychiatry. 2008;65(7):795–803.

Chapter 28
Thrombocytopenia

A platelet count of <150,000 cells/μL is considered thrombocytopenia. However, 2.5% of the population has counts less than this cutoff.

Thrombocytopenia	Platelet count (cells/μL)
Mild	100,000–150,000
Moderate	50,000–100,000
Severe	<50,000

Pathology

Thrombocytopenia is caused by deficient production in the bone marrow, immune-mediated peripheral destruction, or increased sequestration in the spleen.

Etiology

Causes other than psychotropic agents are listed as follows.

Common conditions associated with thrombocytopenia

Nonpsychotropic drugs (antibiotics, cardiac medications, nonsteroidal anti-inflammatory agents)
Chronic infections—HIV, Hepatitis C
Chronic liver disease
Chronic alcohol use
Nutritional deficiencies (Vit B12, folate)
Idiopathic thrombocytopenic purpura (ITP)

© Springer International Publishing AG 2017

189

A. Annamalai, *Medical Management of Psychotropic Side Effects*,
DOI 10.1007/978-3-319-51026-2_28

Psychotropic Medications and Thrombocytopenia

Drug-induced thrombocytopenia is usually mediated by immune mechanisms, namely, platelet destruction by platelet reactive antibodies. Bone marrow suppression is a less common cause of isolated drug-induced thrombocytopenia.

Psychotropic-induced thrombocytopenia is reported only in a small minority of cases. If it is moderate or severe, it is likely to be associated with leukopenia or anemia. Some known offending agents are valproate (medicated by bone marrow suppression) and carbamazepine (platelet destruction that is independent of its effect on bone marrow suppression). Almost any psychotropic agent can cause thrombocytopenia [1] but there are only rare reports of bleeding resulting from psychotropic medications [2].

Generally, drug-induced thrombocytopenia occurs with 1 week of treatment initiation. Recovery of platelets occurs within 5–7 days of stopping an offending medication.

> ***Thrombocytopenia from psychotropic medications is usually mild; if medication is stopped, it reverses within days.***

Clinical Features

Bleeding risk increases with severity of thrombocytopenia. Initial signs seen with mild reduction in platelets are easy skin bruising and mucosal bleeding. There is no safe level of platelet count as bleeding risk depends on individual factors. But generally surgical bleeding risk increases only in severe thrombocytopenia and spontaneous hemorrhagic bleeding occurs at counts $<20,000/\mu L$

> ***Easy skin bruising and mucosal bleeding are the most likely complications of drug-induced thrombocytopenia; even these symptoms are generally not seen until the thrombocytopenia is moderate to severe.***

Diagnosis

There is no need to perform coagulation studies unless thrombocytopenia is severe. If the platelet count is indeed extremely low, patients should be referred for workup of nondrug etiologies. Laboratory testing for drug-dependent antiplatelet antibodies exist but are not easily available and not necessary in evaluation of drug-induced thrombocytopenia.

There is no need to do any testing to establish medications as cause for thrombocytopenia.

Patients with severe thrombocytopenia should be referred for workup of other etiologies.

Management

There is no need to monitor platelet counts on any psychotropic medication. The temporal relationship between the drug and onset of thrombocytopenia is important in establishing the cause. Other common causes encountered in psychiatric patients should be considered as contributing factors. When the diagnosis is uncertain, temporarily stopping the drug can be a useful strategy. However, if thrombocytopenia is mild, this is unnecessary. Drug-induced thrombocytopenia is almost never severe enough to require discontinuing medication unless accompanied by other blood dyscrasias.

There is no need to monitor platelet counts during psychotropic treatment.

In rare cases of moderate or severe thrombocytopenia, medication should be stopped.

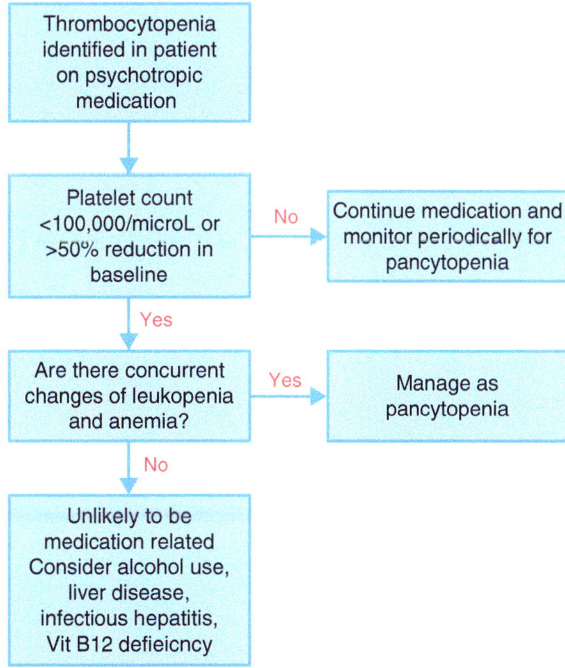

References

1. Oyesanmi O, Kunkel EJ, Monti DA, Field HL. Hematologic side effects of psychotropics. Psychosomatics. 1999;40(5):414–21.
2. Stubner S, Grohmann R, Engel R, Bandelow B, Ludwig WD, Wagner G, et al. Blood dyscrasias induced by psychotropic drugs. Pharmacopsychiatry. 2004;37(Suppl 1):S70–8.

Chapter 29
Anemia

Anemia is defined as a reduction in red blood counts, hemoglobin, and hematocrit. The latter two parameters are generally used in diagnosing anemia. Prevalence varies with age and can be >10% in older adults.

Definition of anemia

	Hemoglobin (g/dL)	Hematocrit (%)
Men	<13.5	<41
Women	<12	<36

The normal ranges for hemoglobin and hematocrit may be different from the previous values depending on country of origin, race, living altitude, physical activity level, and smoking status.

Pathology

Anemia results from decreased red blood cell production in the bone marrow, increased peripheral destruction, or blood loss. Anemia results in clinical symptoms due to reduced oxygen carrying capacity of blood to peripheral tissues.

Many red cell indices are used to assess anemia. Among them, mean corpuscular volume (MCV) is a measure of the average red blood cell size. Reticulocyte count is the percentage of immature red blood cells and is a measure of red blood cell production by the bone marrow.

© Springer International Publishing AG 2017

A. Annamalai, *Medical Management of Psychotropic Side Effects*,

DOI 10.1007/978-3-319-51026-2_29

Etiology

Decreased red blood cell production can be from bone marrow disorders or nutritional deficiencies (iron, vitamin B12, folate). Morphologic abnormalities like thalassemia cause ineffective red blood cell formation. Increased destruction occurs in various hemolytic anemias and conditions causing an enlarged spleen. Many chronic diseases cause anemia by various mechanisms.

Psychotropic Medications and Anemia

Many medications cause anemia by immune-mediated hemolysis. The mechanism of psychotropic-induced anemia may be similar, but red blood cell aplasia has also been reported [1]. Anemia thought to result from a medication usually does not need any intervention. Isolated psychotropic-induced anemia is rare and almost never severe enough to warrant any diagnostic workup or stopping the medication. Since anemia associated with psychotropic medications is generally not clinically significant, not much is known about characteristics of the anemia.

Anemia can occasionally be a concern with psychotropic drug treatment when it occurs as part of a pancytopenia. This is discussed in Chapter 30. See the following table for list of psychotropic medications that have been reported to cause anemia [1, 2].

Anemia and psychotropic agents

Usually associated with pancytopenia	Carbamazepine, mirtazapine
Isolated anemia	Lamotrigine, some selective serotonin reuptake inhibitors, venlafaxine

Isolated anemia from psychotropic medications almost never is significant enough to require intervention.

Clinical Features

Generally, symptoms related to anemia occur gradually and include fatigue, exertional dyspnea, and palpitations. Chronic persistent severe anemia can cause serious complications such as cardiomyopathy.

If anemia results from psychotropic medications, it usually occurs in the first 2 months of treatment.

Anemia is commonly associated with fatigue.

Diagnosis

Among the red blood cell indices, MCV is frequently used to evaluate the cause of anemia. It is low in iron deficiency anemia, thalassemias, and high with ethanol abuse, folate, and vitamin B12 deficiency. If more than one cause of anemia is present, MCV may be normal. Reticulocyte count is high in situations of increased red cell destruction such as hemolysis and acute blood loss.

Macrocytic anemia (high MCV) and red cell aplasia (low reticulocyte count) are both described with lamotrigine. There is no distinguishing characteristic that can be attributed to anemia from psychotropic medications.

> *MCV and reticulocyte count are two key indices to differentiate etiology of anemia.*
>
> *Anemia due to psychotropic medications does not have unique distinguishing characteristics.*

The table lists common etiologies and associated changes in red cell indices.

Abnormalities associated with common etiologies of anemia

Acute blood loss	Normal MCV, increased reticulocyte count
Iron deficiency anemia	Low MCV, low reticulocyte count, low serum iron and ferritin, high iron binding capacity
Anemia of chronic disease	Normal MCV, low to normal reticulocyte count, low iron and low iron binding capacity
Alcohol abuse, folate, and vitamin B12 deficiencies	High MCV, low to normal reticulocyte count, low serum B12 or folate
Hemolytic anemia	Increased reticulocytes, low haptoglobin, increased lactate dehydrogenase, bilirubin

Management

If anemia is detected, patient should be evaluated for common etiologies. Lab indices cannot be used to reliably identify drug-induced anemia. But other previously undiagnosed anemias should be detected and treated. A detailed history including chronology of anemia and timing of start of offending medication may help to identify anemia from medications. An isolated asymptomatic mild anemia due to a medication does not need any intervention. Unless the anemia is severe, long-term complications from chronic anemia are unlikely.

> *Common etiologies of anemia should be identified and treated.*
>
> *Isolated anemia from medications is usually mild and has no long-term sequelae.*

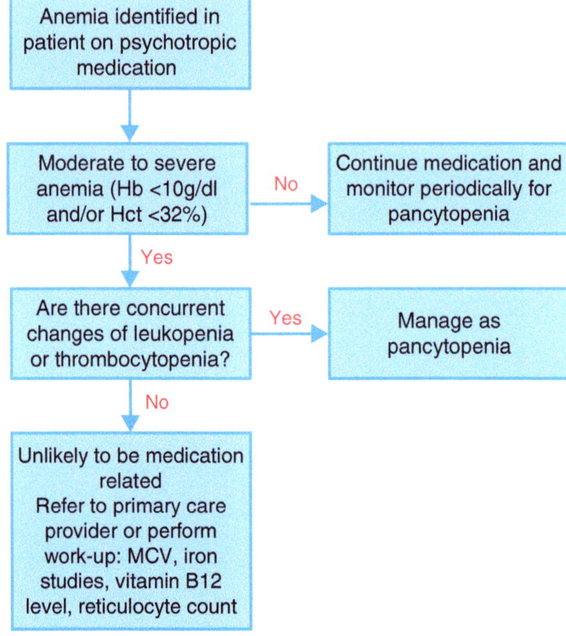

References

1. Esfahani FE, Dasheiff RM. Anemia associated with lamotrigine. Neurology. 1997;49(1):306–7.
2. Oyesanmi O, Kunkel EJ, Monti DA, Field HL. Hematologic side effects of psychotropics. Psychosomatics. 1999;40(5):414–21.

Chapter 30
Pancytopenia

It is defined as a decrease in all blood cell lines resulting in anemia, neutropenia, and thrombocytopenia.

Pathology

There is a deficiency of hematopoietic stem cells in the bone marrow due to direct toxicity by external agents, immune destruction of stem cells, or bone marrow replacement by malignancy or fibrosis. Rarely, pancytopenia is congenital.

Etiology

Acquired pancytopenia is due to drugs (sulfonamides, anticonvulsants), viral infections, and autoimmune disease. It is an expected side effect of chemotherapeutic treatment.

Psychotropic Medications and Pancytopenia

It is an extremely rare idiosyncratic reaction to psychotropic agents [1]. There are case reports with carbamazepine, valproate, olanzapine, and clozapine.

When it does occur, it can be severe and life threatening. It can be seen within a few days of starting the medication. Stopping the medication rapidly brings the blood counts back to normal.

> *Psychotropic medication-induced pancytopenia is extremely rare; when it occurs it usually reverses soon after stopping the medication.*

© Springer International Publishing AG 2017

A. Annamalai, *Medical Management of Psychotropic Side Effects*,
DOI 10.1007/978-3-319-51026-2_30

Clinical Features

Symptoms may include fatigue, pallor, tachycardia, bleeding, infection, and fever.

> ***Symptoms related to reduced counts of all cell lines may develop over days or occur more acutely.***

Diagnosis

Pancytopenia is diagnosed when there is a decrease in all three cell lines. A bone marrow aspiration and biopsy may be necessary if aplastic anemia with bone marrow aplasia is suspected. Diagnosis of medication-induced pancytopenia depends on the temporal relationship of dyscrasia occurrence and medication initiation.

> ***Additional testing is only required to rule out other etiologies as when diagnosis is uncertain or when the dyscrasias do not resolve with stopping the medication.***

Management

Psychotropic medications cause pancytopenia infrequently and so routine monitoring is not required unless the medication requires monitoring for leukopenia (e.g., clozapine). Lab testing usually is in response to clinical symptoms, at which time the cytopenia is likely to be at least moderate in severity. Any patient who develops pancytopenia needs immediate treatment even if pancytopenia is mild as it can progress rapidly. If a medication is suspected as the cause it should immediately be stopped. The blood counts will revert to normal in a matter of days once the causative agent is removed.

In severe cases of pancytopenia, other treatments such as blood transfusion, granulocyte-stimulating factor, and corticosteroids may be needed.

> ***Pancytopenia occurs very rarely with psychotropic medications; when it does, medication should be stopped immediately even if the cytopenia is mild.***

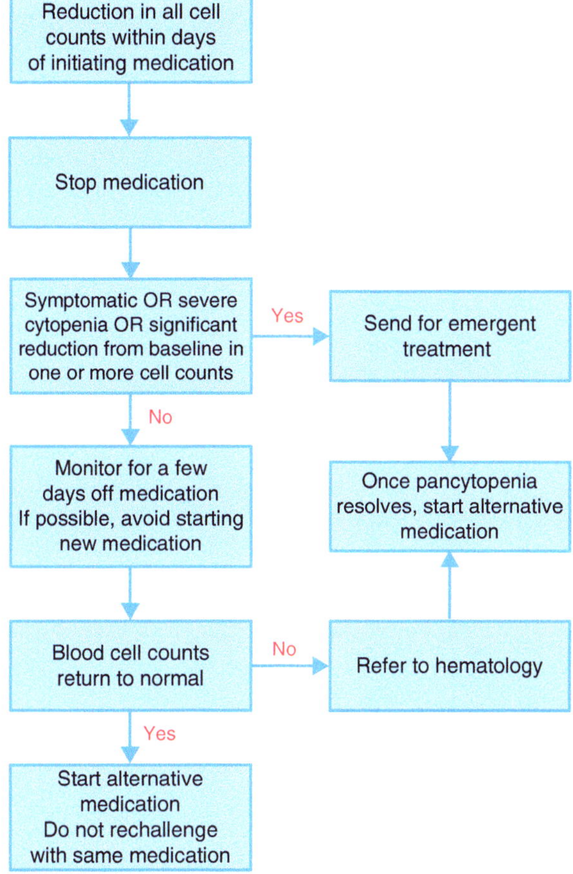

Reference

1. Stubner S, Grohmann R, Engel R, Bandelow B, Ludwig WD, Wagner G, et al. Blood dyscrasias induced by psychotropic drugs. Pharmacopsychiatry. 2004;37(Suppl 1):S70–8.

Chapter 31
Leukocytosis

Leukocytosis can be due to increase in any of the white blood cell (WBC) counts but commonly is due to an increase in neutrophils. Neutrophilia is used interchangeably with leukocytosis.

Pathology

Leukocytosis is due to increased production of WBCs or increased release of WBCs from bone marrow or blood vessels where many WBCS are stored.

Etiology

Leukocytosis is commonly seen in infections, physical or emotional stress, and medications (steroids). It can be seen in chronic heavy smokers. A less common cause is a primary hematologic malignancy. Some patients with chronic idiopathic neutrophilia have WBCs outside the normal range with no identified cause.

Psychotropic Medications and Leukocytosis

Lithium causes an increase in neutrophils leading to neutrophilia and leukocytosis. It is due to both margination of cells into the periphery as well as a direct action of lithium on the bone marrow. The white blood cell (WBC) counts increase, on average, by 2500 cells/μL. It starts with a week of treatment and persists chronically [1]. The WBC typically does not rise above 20,000 cells/μL. Lithium-induced leukocytosis

© Springer International Publishing AG 2017

A. Annamalai, *Medical Management of Psychotropic Side Effects*,
DOI 10.1007/978-3-319-51026-2_31

generally requires no intervention. The leukocytosis is sometimes accompanied by thrombocytosis.

Antipsychotics including clozapine can cause a small degree of leukocytosis. Carbamazepine can occasionally cause leukocytosis [2].

> *Neutrophilia caused by lithium is rarely >20,000 cells/μL.*

Clinical Features

Leukocytosis from lithium has no associated symptoms. Symptoms of leukocytosis from other etiologies will reflect the underlying cause of the elevated WBC count. An infectious process will cause fever and symptoms corresponding to the source of infection.

> *Any symptom seen with neutrophilia is that of the underlying disease process, if any.*

Diagnosis

A WBC count >11,000 cells/μL is usually the cutoff for an abnormal count. But people can have WBCs in the 11,000–40,000 range with no identified pathology. A WBC count >50,000 cells/μL is considered hyperleukocytosis.

A WBC differential will determine if leukocytosis is from neutrophilia or an increase in other WBC lines. Coexisting anemia and increased platelet count may indicate chronic infection or inflammation. A peripheral smear can identify immature WBCs and possibly a hematologic malignancy. A bone marrow evaluation is rarely necessary unless a primary hematologic malignancy is suspected.

> *Isolated leukocytosis from lithium does not require any additional testing except to rule out other nonmedication causes.*

Management

There is no need to monitor WBC count during lithium treatment. If leukocytosis is detected while on lithium, no intervention is required. Lithium can be continued without additional monitoring. However, when leukocytosis is identified, it should not be presumed to result from treatment with lithium, especially if the increase in WBCs is >2500 cells/μL from baseline or total WBC count is >20,000 cells/μL.

Other etiologies such as bacterial infections, steroid therapy, strenuous trauma, and severe stress should be considered.

The leukocytosis from lithium can sometimes exceed 20,000 cells/µL but this value can be used as a threshold to consider hematology referral. The referral is only needed if the leukocytosis is persistent and no other etiology is identified.

Lithium can be continued with leukocytosis.

A hematology referral can be considered if WBC is persistently >20,000 cells/µL.

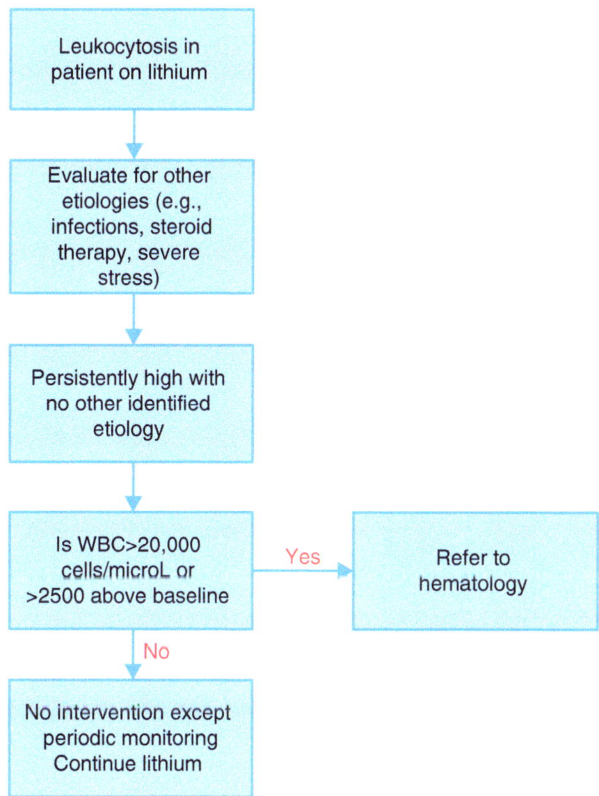

References

1. Carmen J, Okafor K, Ike E. The effects of lithium therapy on leukocytes: a 1-year follow-up study. J Natl Med Assoc. 1993;85(4):301–3.
2. Flanagan RJ, Dunk L. Haematological toxicity of drugs used in psychiatry. Hum Psychopharmacol. 2008;23(Suppl 1):27–41.

Chapter 32
Eosinophilia

Eosinophilia refers to an absolute eosinophil count >500 cells/μL. A value >5000 cells/μL is considered severe eosinophilia.

Pathology

Eosinophils are primarily seen in tissues and are much less abundant in peripheral blood. The clinical significance of eosinophilia is the potential for organ damage with high eosinophil levels.

Etiology

Major causes are atopic disease, medication allergies, and parasitic infections. Less commonly, primary hematologic disorders cause elevations in eosinophils.

Psychotropic Medications and Eosinophilia

Eosinophilia caused by psychotropic medications is usually mild, transient, and benign. It usually occurs early in treatment. Various mechanisms including a type of hypersensitivity reaction has been proposed. Tricyclic antidepressants, some typical antipsychotics and clozapine cause mild eosinophilia [1, 2]. The eosinophilia rarely causes eosinophilic end organ damage. There are case reports of clozapine-related eosinophilic colitis, pleural effusion, and pancreatitis. Eosinophilia is often a feature of clozapine-induced myocarditis. There are also reports of eosinophilic pulmonary complications from serotonin reuptake inhibitors [3]. Eosinophilia can also be seen

© Springer International Publishing AG 2017
A. Annamalai, *Medical Management of Psychotropic Side Effects*,
DOI 10.1007/978-3-319-51026-2_32

as part of a syndrome of Drug Reaction with Eosinophila and Systemic Syndromes (DRESS). Features of DRESS syndrome are described in Chapter 33.

> ***Psychotropic medications usually cause transient and benign eosinophilia; they rarely result in eosinophilic end organ damage.***

Clinical Features

Symptoms are usually limited to the underlying cause of eosinophilia. If related to medication exposure, it may be asymptomatic or present with skin allergy as in DRESS. If end organ infiltration has occurred, symptoms specific to that organ dysfunction will be seen.

> ***Medication-induced eosinophilia is not symptomatic unless end organ infiltration has occurred.***

Diagnosis

A complete blood count and peripheral smear should be performed as initial tests to look for coexistent blood dyscrasias. For isolated eosinophilia, environmental exposures and infections should be ruled out by clinical and lab evaluation. In a patient with eosinophilia and symptoms of organ dysfunction, biopsy of the relevant organ should be considered. The biopsy will show eosinophilic infiltration. In persistent severe eosinophilia with no identified etiology, a referral for possible marrow evaluation can be considered.

> ***In medication-induced eosinophilic end organ damage, biopsy will show eosinophilic infiltration.***

Management

There is no need to monitor eosinophil counts on any psychotropic medication. Psychotropic drug-induced eosinophilia is most likely to be identified on routine lab monitoring. There is no cutoff for eosinophil count that can accurately predict risk for serious complications. Unless there is any evidence of end organ damage or a serious systemic reaction like DRESS, there is no need to interrupt or stop the psychotropic medication.

If a medication is stopped, it should be noted that eosinophil count might take weeks to months to return to normal. Hence, stopping the medication cannot immediately be used as a diagnostic tool to definitively establish medication as the cause for eosinophilic complications. If severe eosinophilia develops when patient is on a psychotropic medication, it is prudent to switch the medication, especially if the dyscrasia occurred in the early phase of treatment.

During psychotropic treatment, if eosinophilia occurs and is severe or accompanied by additional symptoms, medication should be stopped if no other etiology is identified.

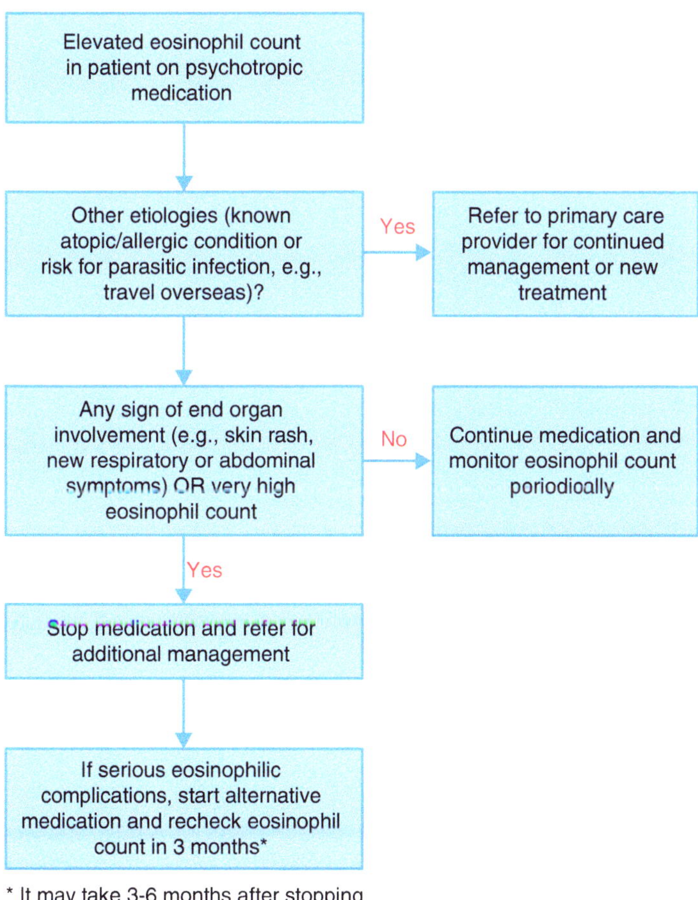

References

1. Flanagan RJ, Dunk L. Haematological toxicity of drugs used in psychiatry. Hum Psychopharmacol. 2008;23(Suppl 1):27–41.
2. Oyesanmi O, Kunkel EJ, Monti DA, Field HL. Hematologic side effects of psychotropics. Psychosomatics. 1999;40(5):414–21.
3. Thornton C, Maher TM, Hansell D, Nicholson AG, Wells AU. Pulmonary fibrosis associated with psychotropic drug therapy: a case report. J Med Case Reports. 2009;3:126.

Section IX
Dermatology

Chapter 33
Drug-Induced Cutaneous Reactions

Cutaneous reactions are a common adverse effect of medications. Most are mild but some can be serious and require drug discontinuation.

Pathology

Most drug-induced skin reactions are immune mediated.

Etiology

Almost any medication can cause an allergic skin reaction. Common offenders for serious reactions are antibiotics, anticonvulsants, and anticoagulants.

Psychotropic Medications and Skin Reactions

Many psychotropic medications have the potential to cause a skin allergy. Common types are exanthematous eruptions (diffuse red macules or papules) and urticarial rashes (itchy red plaques). Almost any medication can cause these benign skin reactions but some medication classes are more commonly implicated. For example, phenothiazines are associated with exanthems and tricyclic antidepressants (TCAs) are associated with urticaria [1]. Serious skin reactions associated with anticonvulsants are Stevens–Johnson syndrome (SJS) and Toxic Epidermal Necrolysis (TEN), different stages of a necrolytic syndrome with high mortality.

© Springer International Publishing AG 2017
A. Annamalai, *Medical Management of Psychotropic Side Effects*,
DOI 10.1007/978-3-319-51026-2_33

Most medication-induced skin rashes are benign and resolve on stopping the medication; common rashes are exanthems and urticaria.

Most skin reactions are dose dependent and resolve when the medication is stopped. Onset is usually within hours to days after exposure but can occur at any time. There may be cross-reactivity between drugs within the same class and this should be a consideration especially with serious reactions.

Most medication-induced skin reactions are dose dependent and reversible upon stopping the medication.

See table for skin reactions commonly associated with particular medication classes.

Psychotropic medications and associated skin lesions [1]

Drug/class	Associated skin reaction	
Carbamazepine, lamotrigine	Erythema multiforme	Well-defined macules or papules with distinct color zones
	Lichenoid reaction	Violaceous flat-topped papules usually on trunk
	SJS/TEN	Diffuse, spreading rash involving mucous membranes causing eventual sloughing of skin
	DRESS	Maculopapular spreading rash often with facial edema
Phenothiazines (and less commonly other antipsychotics)	Photosensivity/photopigmentation	Skin changes in sun exposed areas
	Exanthematous eruptions	Diffuse maculopapular eruptions, itchy
Lithium	Hair loss	Usually from scalp, diffuse
	Acneiform eruptions	Reddish papules, pustules on skin follicles
	Psoriasis	New onset or exacerbation
Valproate	Hair loss	Usually from scalp, diffuse
	Pseudolymphoma	Red or violaceous papules, plaques or nodules, itchy

Drug/class	Associated skin reaction	
SSRIs, SNRIs	Hyperhidrosis	Increased sweating especially in palms
	Exanthematous eruptions	Diffuse maculopapular eruptions, itchy
	Urticaria	Raised areas of erythema, itchy
TCAs	Angioedema	Skin swelling, usually around eyes and lips
	Urticaria	Raised areas of erythema, itchy
Benzodiazepines	Photosensitivity	Skin changes in sun exposed areas
	Pseudolymphoma	Red or violaceous papules, plaques or nodules, itchy

Note: While the lesions listed above are associated with these agents, the incidence for most skin reactions is low

Psychotropic medications associated with SJS/TEN are carbamazepine and lamotrigine [1]. While these medications are the causative agents in a large majority of people with SJS/TEN, the absolute risk is small. It is <1% with carbamazepine and <0.05% with lamotrigine. There are rare case reports associated with oxcarbazepine and valproate. The combination of valproate and lamotrigine significantly increases the risk. Risk with lamotrigine can be reduced by slow titration and the same strategy may work for carbamazepine too [1]. People of certain ethnicity and with particular genotypes are at higher risk for this syndrome. Women appear at higher risk and this may be related to a higher risk of autoimmune disorders.

The absolute risk of a serious necrolytic syndrome with carbamazepine and lamotrigine is small.

See table for features of SJS/TEN.

Stevens–Johnson syndrome

Severe mucocutaneous reaction caused usually by medications
Pathology: Cell-mediated toxic reaction against skin cells
Causes: Mostly medications; less commonly, infections, vaccines, contrast dye
Symptoms: Fever, spreading rash (starts in face, mucous membrane involved, sometimes bullous, easy sloughing of skin); onset within days of exposure; when a large surface area is involved, it is termed toxic epidermal necrolysis
Lab findings: Cytopenias, electrolyte imbalance related to fluid loss
Management: Withdrawal of triggering agent; supportive care as in severe third degree burns
Prognosis: More than 25% mortality (from sepsis and organ failure as in severe burn injury)

A less well-known skin reaction is Drug Rash with Eosinophilia and Systemic Syndromes (DRESS), a potentially fatal hypersensitivity reaction [2].

Carbamazepine, lamotrigine, and valproate are the medications implicated in this syndrome also. DRESS is difficult to recognize as skin changes and other symptoms are nonspecific and onset is usually some weeks after exposure. See table for features of DRESS.

DRESS syndrome

Drug-induced hypersensitivity reaction that involves skin eruptions, hematologic abnormalities, and internal organ damage
Pathology: Drug specific immune response;
Causes: By definition, medications; onset is 2–6 weeks after exposure
Symptoms: Starts as diffuse spreading rash (erythematous, usually not raised); followed by fever, facial edema, lymph node enlargement, symptoms of other organ involvement
Lab findings: Elevated eosinophil and lymphocyte counts; signs of liver or kidney damage
Management: Withdrawal of offending medication and supportive care
Prognosis: Less than 10% mortality rate (usually from hepatic necrosis)

While lamotrigine and carbamazepine are associated with many cases of SJS/TEN and DRESS, clinicians should remember that they are more likely to cause benign rashes.

Clinical Features

Skin rash from drugs can take on many forms as previously described. The most common allergy, drug exanthem looks like red, flat, diffusely spread lesions over chest, back, or upper extremities that coalesce in some areas. The lesions are often itchy.

A benign skin rash may not be easily distinguishable from one that will progress to a serious syndrome. A skin rash that is extensive, continues to spread, and associated with systemic symptoms may herald progression to more serious syndromes. In SJS, the rash usually starts in the face and mucous membranes are involved; initially it may be flat and red but then can become raised, fluid filled, and crusted. In later stages of SJS, as it progresses to TEN, the superficial skin layer easily sloughs off. In DRESS, facial edema is often seen in the early stages.

Any skin rash that starts in the face, involves mucous membranes or is associated with systemic symptoms should be treated as a potential harbinger of a serious complication like SJS/TEN.

Diagnosis

The diagnosis of a drug-induced skin rash can only be made based on chronology of rash and medication exposure as well as resolution following drug withdrawal. Other common etiologies such as tinea (lesion with central clearing and raised borders), localized allergy to irritants (usually redness with itching), herpes zoster (starts as red raised lesions that become fluid filled; usually confined to single dermatomal area) are usually easily identified if present.

Patient with certain Human Leukocyte Antigen (HLA) alleles are at higher risk for developing SJS/TEN. Lab testing is not routinely done in clinical practice. Some experts recommend testing in certain ethnicities (Asian) with a higher risk for this genetic association, before starting carbamazepine.

> *The characteristics of the rash help rule out infectious and other allergic etiologies; but the only way to definitively diagnose a medication-induced skin rash is onset after exposure and resolution after stopping medication.*

Management

Drug rash is commonly mild and transient and often needs no intervention. In general, if patient has a localized rash with no systemic symptoms, medication can be continued with careful monitoring. If patient has a progressively spreading rash, it is advisable to stop any medication to prevent potential serious complications. If mucous membranes are involved, the medication should definitely be stopped.

In the case of lamotrigine, carbamazepine, or other anticonvulsants, it is advisable to stop the medication and monitor even when rash is localized with no systemic manifestations. There should be a low threshold for stopping lamotrigine and carbamazepine. If the rash is benign and resolves with stopping the medication, the medication can be cautiously tried again with even slower titration if possible. If the rash is extensive or either SJS/TEN or DRESS occurs, the medication should not ever be attempted again. Due to potential for cross-reactivity between agents of the same class, an alternative medication from a different class is prudent after a severe systemic reaction to a medication.

Prevention is key and it is important to reduce risk of rash occurrence by slow medication titration for high-risk medications such as carbamazepine and lamotrigine. If these medications are stopped for any reason and restarted after a gap of approximately 5 days, they should be slowly titrated again.

Medications can be continued and patient monitored if rash is mild and localized unless the medication is carbamazepine or lamotrigine.

Any rash that does not resolve with continued monitoring warrants stopping the medication.

After a serious drug reaction, medication should never be attempted; an alternative agent from a different class should preferably be used.

Drugs with potential for serious skin reaction should be titrated up slowly.

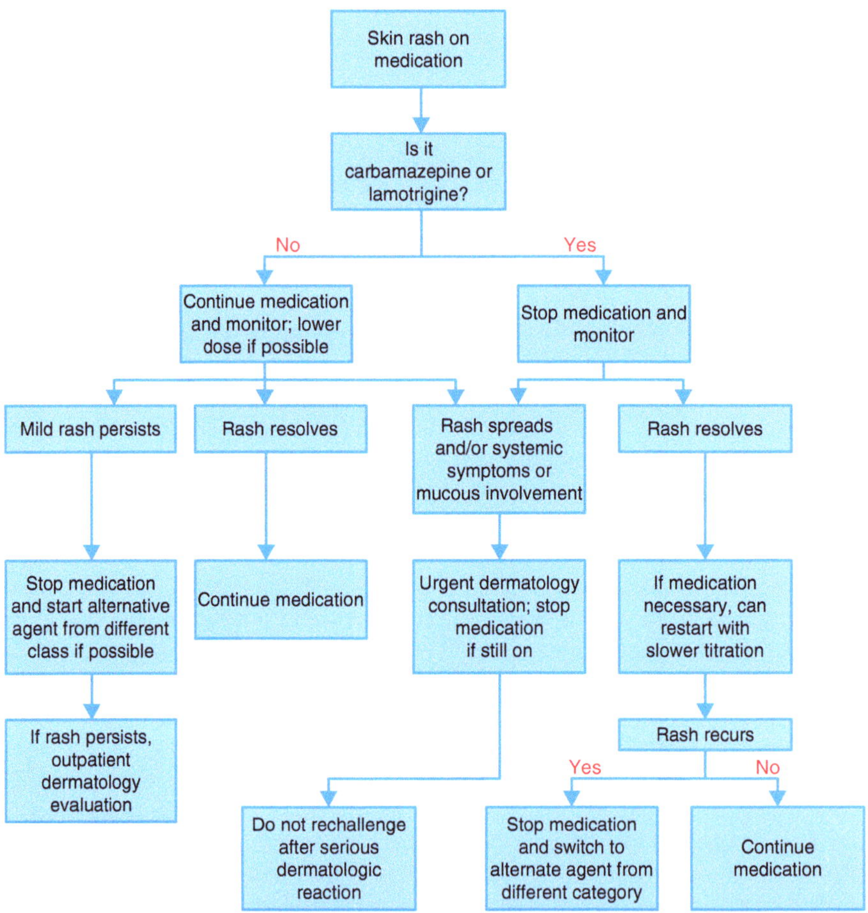

References

1. Mitkov MV, Trowbridge RM, Lockshin BN, Caplan JP. Dermatologic side effects of psychotropic medications. Psychosomatics. 2014;55(1):1–20.
2. Bommersbach TJ, Lapid MI, Leung JG, Cunningham JL, Rummans TA, Kung S. Management of psychotropic drug-induced DRESS syndrome: a systematic review. Mayo Clin Proc. 2016;91(6):787–801.

Section X
Neurologic System
Movement Disorders

Chapter 34
Introduction to Movement Disorders

Movement disorders refer to any disruption of voluntary movement including involuntary muscle activity, though often people use the term to refer to extrapyramidal syndromes caused by antipsychotics.

Movement disorders can be classified broadly as hyperkinetic and hypokinetic disorders based on the characteristics of the involuntary muscle activity.

Pathology

Movement disorders can result from any disruption of the interaction between the pyramidal tracts, basal ganglia, and cerebellum. Most are caused by disorders of the basal ganglia.

Etiology

Different types of movement disorders with their nonpsychotropic etiologies are listed in the table. Bradykinesia seen in Parkinson disease is an example of a hypokinetic movement. Examples of hyperkinetic movements are tremors, tics, dystonias, akathisia, chorea, athetosis, hemiballismus, and myoclonus.

© Springer International Publishing AG 2017

A. Annamalai, *Medical Management of Psychotropic Side Effects*,

DOI 10.1007/978-3-319-51026-2_34

Types of movement disorders and etiologic conditions

Abnormal movement	Characteristic	Causes (nonpsychotropic)
Tremor	Regular, rhythmic, oscillatory	Stress, caffeine, alcohol intoxication and withdrawal, medications (e.g., beta agonist inhalers), familial, Parkinson disease, cerebellar degeneration
Tics	Nonrhythmic, rapid, stereotypical, repetitive; motor or phonatory; difficult to suppress	Tourette syndrome, Huntington disease, infections, stimulant use, cocaine
Dystonias	Sustained contractions sometimes accompanied by repetitive movements	Cerebral palsy, multiple sclerosis, degenerative disorders
Myoclonus	Rapid, jerky twitches, nonsuppressible; may be focal or generalized	Systemic metabolic abnormalities, encephalitis, hypoxia, dementias, medication toxicity
Hemiballismus	Nonrhythmic, rapid, flinging, nonsuppressible	Stroke in subthalamic nucleus
Chorea	Nonrhythmic, jerky, rapid, nonsuppressible; usually in distal muscles or face	Huntington disease, autoimmune disorders, severe hyperthyroidism, central nervous system lupus
Athetosis	Nonrhythmic, slow, writhing, flowing	Hepatic encephalopathy, Huntington disease, encephalitis, cocaine
Akathisia	Subjective and objective motor restlessness	Agitation seen in psychosis or delirium may resemble akathisia
Tardive dyskinesia	Involuntary movements of face, trunk, extremities that occurs after prolonged exposure to triggering agent; can be dystonia, akathisia, tremor	Long-term treatment with dopamine blocking agents (antiemetics, antihistamines, estrogen supplements)

Psychotropic Medications and Movement Disorders

Medications can cause a range of movement abnormalities at toxic doses. There are also specific movement disorders associated with long-term use of some psychotropic medications. They are summarized in the table and described in subsequent chapters.

Movement disorders associated with psychotropic medications

Tremor	Mood stabilizers
	Tricyclic antidepressants
	Serotonin reuptake inhibitors
	Antipsychotics
Extrapyramidal symptoms (dystonia, akathisia, tardive dyskinesia)	Antipsychotics
Tics	Stimulants
Myoclonus (with serotonin syndrome)	Serotonin reuptake inhibitors, tricyclic antidepressants, lithium

Choreoathetosis and hemiballismus are caused by neurologic disorders and are not further discussed. However, movements of tardive dyskinesia may have features of choreoathetosis.

Chapter 35
Tremor

Tremors are involuntary rhythmic oscillatory movements of one or more muscle groups. They most commonly affect the hands but can also involve the legs, face, and trunk.

Pathology

Tremor results from functional hyperexcitability of neuronal loops (mainly through basal ganglia and cerebellum) and structural pathology via neurodegeneration. It can result from lesions in the brainstem, extrapyramidal system, and cerebellum or neurologic injury from ischemia, metabolic disorders, and neurodegenerative diseases.

Medications cause tremors by either exacerbating an underlying physiologic tremor or inducing excitability in muscle receptors and neuronal reflexes.

Etiology

Physiologic tremor occurs in normal individuals and is evident only when exacerbated by stress, sleep deprivation, medications, or substances. Agents that exacerbate tremor include nicotine, caffeine, alcohol, stimulants, benzodiazepine withdrawal, thyroid supplements, and beta agonist inhalers. Essential tremor, often familial, is clinically impairing and may also exacerbate with stress. This tremor is diagnosed when no other etiologies are identified. A psychogenic tremor is diagnosed when no etiology is identified and tremor has certain characteristics. Disease conditions that cause any type of neurologic injury can result in tremors. Tremor is a common symptom in Parkinson disease and cerebellar degeneration. Wilson disease is a rare systemic disease that often presents with tremor.

© Springer International Publishing AG 2017

A. Annamalai, *Medical Management of Psychotropic Side Effects*,

DOI 10.1007/978-3-319-51026-2_35

Psychotropic Medications and Tremor

Mood stabilizers and antidepressants cause a fine, bilateral, symmetric, dose-related tremor [1]. It usually occurs early in treatment though can develop later. Risk factors are older age and personal or family history of tremors. The tremor sometimes improves with time but usually it is necessary to treat the tremor or stop the offending medication. Among mood stabilizers, prevalence of tremor is lithium > valproate > lamotrigine. Both tricyclic antidepressants and serotonin reuptake inhibitors cause tremors on higher doses, during withdrawal or as a precursor to serious side effects such as serotonin syndrome.

Antipsychotics can cause tremor without other features of parkinsonism. The tremor may be a bilateral action tremor that occurs early in treatment or a tardive tremor that occurs after long-term treatment. Tremor can also be seen along with dystonia and tardive dyskinesia.

The characteristics of tremor associated with different classes of psychotropic medications are described in the table. Also described are features of rest and action tremors.

Characteristics of psychotropic induced tremor

Mood stabilizers	Fine, bilateral, rest tremor; often looks like an exaggerated physiologic tremor
Lithium>valproate>lamotrigine	
Antidepressants	Fine, bilateral, rest tremor; often looks like an exaggerated physiologic tremor
Tricyclic antidepressants, serotonin reuptake inhibitors	
Antipsychotics	Bilateral, early or tardive, action tremor; or rest tremor due to drug-induced parkinsonism

Tremor types

Type	Characteristic
Rest	Occurs when affected body part is supported; diminishes with voluntary movement
Action	Occurs with voluntary use of a muscle group
Postural action	Present when an action is maintained against gravity
Intention	Produced or exacerbated with a targeted action

Tremor is a common adverse effect seen with many psychotropic medications and may reflect worsening of underlying physiologic tremor.

Clinical Features

Tremor most commonly manifests in the hands but can involve the legs, face, and other body parts.

Medication-induced tremor has no single characteristic. The presentation depends on the medication being used. The tremor usually appears early in treatment.

Tremor may be related to timing of medication but often fluctuates during the day and worsens with motor activity. It may also worsen with stimulants like caffeine.

Medication-induced tremor may not be clearly distinguishable from other tremors. The table in the appendix lists characteristics of tremors seen with some common conditions.

> ***Medication-induced tremor usually occurs early in treatment; there is no single characteristic to distinguish them from other tremors.***

Diagnosis

Diagnosis of the etiology of a tremor is mainly clinical. Imaging is only useful when other conditions like cerebellar damage are suspected.

> ***Onset of tremor with exposure to medication is the only way to diagnose medication-induced tremor.***

Management

When tremor is seen in patients on psychotropic medications, other common etiologies should be ruled out. If medication is the most likely cause of the tremor, then additional agents that worsen tremors should be eliminated if possible. Examples are caffeine, nicotine, substances that cause withdrawal syndromes, stimulant medications, and herbal supplements. Other potentially serious complications such as serotonin syndrome should be ruled out. If the tremor is mild, there is no need to adjust the medication. Sometimes the tremor decreases with time. Reducing the dose of medication may help decrease the tremor. If tremor is disabling, medication may need to be stopped.

With lithium and valproate, changing to a slow release once-daily formulation may help. Toxicity should be ruled out by checking serum levels especially if the tremor characteristic had changed from a fine to a coarse tremor.

Pharmacological treatment can be tried with moderate to severe tremors. Propranolol is a commonly used medication [1]. Primidone shows equivalent efficacy but is not used commonly due to its side effect profile. Benzodiazepines are less efficacious but commonly used. For antipsychotic-induced tremor that is not due to parkinsonism, the same strategies can be tried. There are case reports of olanzapine diminishing tremors when added on to a typical antipsychotic agent [2] but this is not a recommended strategy due to adverse effect profile and polypharmacy.

Eliminating exacerbating factors, changing to extended release formulation, and dose reduction are initial strategies for treating medication-induced tremor.

Mild medication-induced tremor requires no treatment; propranolol may help more severe tremors.

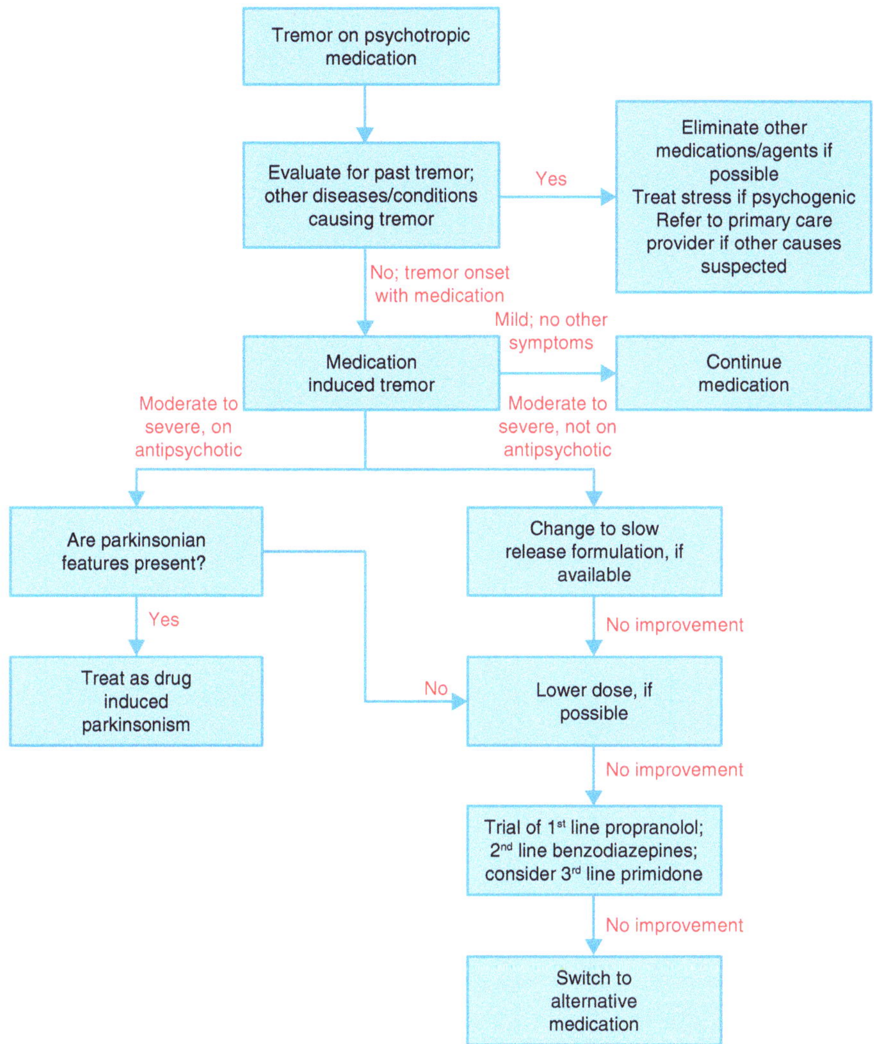
Tremor on psychotropic medication
Evaluate for past tremor; other diseases/conditions causing tremor
Yes
Eliminate other medications/agents if possible
Treat stress if psychogenic
Refer to primary care provider if other causes suspected
No; tremor onset with medication
Medication induced tremor
Mild; no other symptoms
Continue medication
Moderate to severe, on antipsychotic
Moderate to severe, not on antipsychotic
Are parkinsonian features present?
Change to slow release formulation, if available
Yes
No improvement
No
Treat as drug induced parkinsonism
Lower dose, if possible
No improvement
Trial of 1st line propranolol; 2nd line benzodiazepines; consider 3rd line primidone
No improvement
Switch to alternative medication

Appendix

Tremor features in selected disease conditions

Disease condition	Clinical features
Enhanced physiologic tremor	Fine, bilateral, noticeable only with stress or stimulants
Essential tremor	Postural action: generally bilateral, can affect head, voice, starts in young adulthood but brought to clinical attention in later years, responds to alcohol consumption
Parkinson disease	Rest tremor: Low frequency, asymmetric, involves distal extremities
Cerebellar injury/ degeneration	Intention: usually unilateral, other cerebellar signs such as gait imbalance
Psychogenic tremor	Abrupt onset, rest or action, inconsistent and changing features, extinction with distraction, onset possibly with stressor, may be resistant to treatment

References

1. Arbaizar B, Gomez-Acebo I, Llorca J. Postural induced-tremor in psychiatry. Psychiatry Clin Neurosci. 2008;62(6):638–45.
2. Strauss AJ, Bailey RK, Dralle PW, Eschmann AJ, Wagner RB. Conventional psychotropic-induced tremor extinguished by olanzapine. Am J Psychiatry. 1998;155(8):1132.

Chapter 36
Extrapyramidal Symptoms I (Parkinsonism)

Parkinsonism refers to a constellation of symptoms seen in Parkinson disease. Both idiopathic Parkinson disease and other secondary etiologies can cause these symptoms. The predominant symptoms are resting tremor, muscle rigidity, bradykinesia or slowed movements, and postural instability.

Pathology

Dopamine depletion in the basal ganglia leads to motor dysfunction. In Parkinson disease neuronal degeneration is idiopathic. In secondary causes of parkinsonism, the mechanism is interference with dopamine action in the basal ganglia. Dopamine-blocking medications are a common cause of secondary parkinsonism.

Etiology

Besides dopamine-blocking medications, secondary causes of parkinsonism include neurodegenerative disorders (e.g., Lewy body dementia), cerebrovascular disease, tumors (rare), and encephalitis (usually transient).

Psychotropic Medications and Parkinsonism

Drug-induced parkinsonism (DIP) usually occurs within days to weeks after starting antipsychotics though can occur later. There is no clear dose–effect relationship [1]. The tremor is often less prominent than other symptoms of parkinsonism such

© Springer International Publishing AG 2017
A. Annamalai, *Medical Management of Psychotropic Side Effects*,
DOI 10.1007/978-3-319-51026-2_36

as muscle stiffness, bradykinesia, and shuffling gait. As compared to Parkinson disease, the tremor in DIP is more likely to be postural, bilateral, symmetrical, and commonly affects females. Tremor in Parkinson disease occurs at rest, is unilateral, and commonly affects males. But unfortunately, in a large number of cases, DIP presents with features similar to Parkinson disease and the two are not clearly distinguishable. Due to the difficulties in diagnosis, the exact prevalence of DIP is uncertain.

DIP usually resolves within weeks to months of stopping the medication though symptom persistence has been reported [2]. The symptom persistence is reported to be as high as 50% and recurrence of symptoms was reported in 7% patients on long-term follow-up [2]. These cases may reflect underlying Parkinson disease with DIP being a precipitant.

The risk of DIP with different antipsychotic medications correlates with their overall risk of extrapyramidal symptoms. Typical antipsychotics carry a higher risk than atypical agents, though the risk with lower potency typical agents is equivalent to atypical agents. Among atypical antipsychotics, clozapine and quetiapine are the least likely to cause DIP. Even aripiprazole, a partial dopamine agonist, is associated with DIP. Other agents that act by blocking dopamine, such as metoclopramide, can cause DIP. Rarely, lithium, antidepressants, and antiepileptic agents can cause DIP after long-term use due to poorly understood mechanisms.

There is no good evidence for any agent for treatment of DIP. Medications commonly used are anticholinergics (benztropine, trihexyphenidyl), amantadine, and levodopa. Levodopa does not seem to cause significant complications but beneficial effects are also minimal [1].

> ***Antipsychotic-induced parkinsonism is often not distinguishable from Parkinson disease; it does not reverse in all cases after stopping the medication.***
>
> ***Clozapine and quetiapine are least likely to cause this adverse effect.***

Clinical Features

DIP due to antipsychotics occurs relatively early in treatment. In DIP, any feature of parkinsonism like shuffling gait, stooped posture, slowed movements, absence of arm swing, reduced facial expression, or cogwheeling rigidity can be seen. As described earlier, DIP may not be distinguishable from idiopathic Parkinson disease.

> ***Any feature seen in idiopathic Parkinson disease may be seen in drug-induced parkinsonism.***

Diagnosis

Dopamine transporter scans have been suggested as useful for differentiating DIP from Parkinson disease. However, in clinical practice, diagnosis of DIP is made when symptoms of parkinsonism occur early on antipsychotic medications and there is no prior history of Parkinson disease.

> *The diagnosis of drug-induced parkinsonism is made when symptoms appear relatively early during antipsychotic treatment and there is no prior history of Parkinson disease.*

Management

When DIP occurs, medication should be switched to an antipsychotic with lesser propensity for extrapyramidal symptoms, if possible. Clozapine and quetiapine are good choices. Anticholinergics can be tried though there is no good evidence for their efficacy in DIP. Dopaminergic agents can be tried especially if the diagnosis of DIP is in doubt (e.g., if symptoms occur after months to years of antipsychotic treatment) and either antipsychotic medication is important for symptom control or symptoms do not reverse after switching medication. If levodopa is initiated, it should preferably be in conjunction with a neurologist.

> *For drug-induced parkinsonism, medication should preferably be switched; anticholinergics may be tried if medication is continued. Dopaminergic agents can be considered especially when parkinsonism occurs late in treatment.*

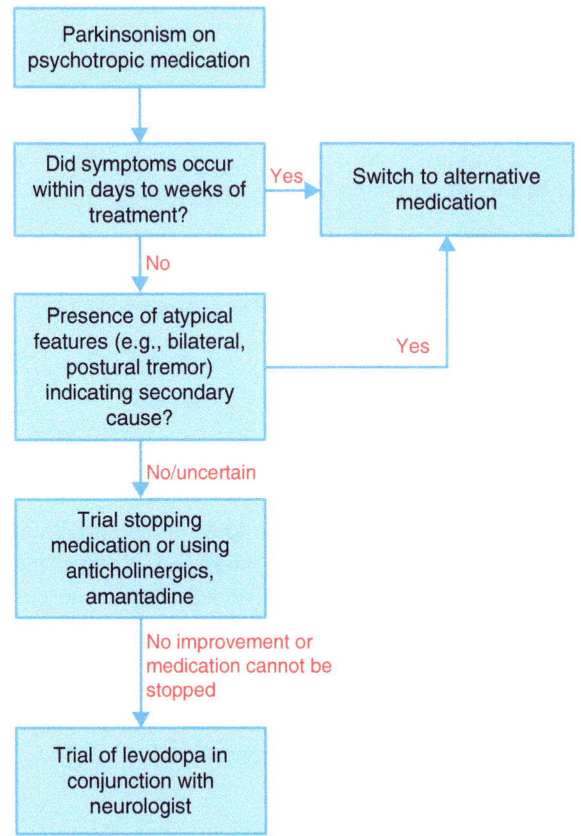

References

1. Hardie RJ, Lees AJ. Neuroleptic-induced Parkinson's syndrome: clinical features and results of treatment with levodopa. J Neurol Neurosurg Psychiatry. 1988;51(6):850–4.
2. Shin HW, Chung SJ. Drug-induced parkinsonism. J Clin Neurol. 2012;8(1):15–21.

Chapter 37
Extrapyramidal Symptoms II (Dystonia, Akathisia, Tardive Dyskinesia)

Extrapyramidal symptoms (EPS) refer to movement disorders that result from lesions in the basal ganglia and its connections, due to interference with dopaminergic transmission. Antipsychotics are a common cause of EPS.

Pathology

The pathology is related to binding and blockade of the dopamine (D2) receptor by the antipsychotic and postsynaptic dopamine receptor supersensitivity. Fluctuations in other neurotransmitters like serotonin and norepinephrine may also contribute to EPS.

Etiology

EPS is caused by dopamine-blocking medications. Antipsychotics are the most common offending agents though other agents like antiemetics with dopamine-blocking effects also cause EPS.

Psychotropic Medications and EPS

Typical antipsychotics are more likely to cause EPS than atypical agents. Higher potency typical antipsychotics are more likely to produce EPS than lower potency typical agents. Low-potency typical antipsychotics and atypical antipsychotics are generally equivalent in their risk though there is variability between different agents [1].

© Springer International Publishing AG 2017

A. Annamalai, *Medical Management of Psychotropic Side Effects*,

DOI 10.1007/978-3-319-51026-2_37

Among atypical agents, risperidone is the most likely and clozapine and quetiapine are the least likely agents to cause EPS.

EPS can be divided into acute and tardive syndromes. There is no uniform consensus on the duration of treatment after which the syndrome is considered tardive but it is usually at least 90 days. More often, the tardive syndromes occur after months or years of treatment. The specific syndromes include dystonia, akathisia, parkinsonism, and tardive dyskinesia. See Chapter 36 for drug-induced parkinsonism. Following is a description of the other three syndromes.

Dystonia

In the absence of preexisting neurodegenerative disorders, medication side effect is the predominant cause of dystonia. The prevalence of acute dystonia from antipsychotics is 10–30%. Ninety percent occur within 5 days of treatment [2]. Mild dystonia usually resolves without treatment. Anticholinergic agents are the mainstay of treatment for acute dystonia. Tardive dystonia is much rarer than acute dystonia. It has a worse prognosis, often persisting after stopping the offending agent. Tardive dystonia may also be seen as part of parkinsonism.

Akathisia

Akathisia is seen in up to 36% people on antipsychotics [2]. It is usually seen within 2 weeks of treatment and 90% occur within 10 weeks. It may be hard to differentiate from agitation secondary to psychotic symptoms, anxiety, substance withdrawal, restless leg syndrome, and acute delirium from metabolic abnormalities. Akathisia has features similar to restless legs syndrome but can usually be differentiated clinically. The latter presents mostly at night or during periods of inactivity; also, it mainly involves the legs and spares other parts of the body. Akathisia may also be seen as part of parkinsonism.

As with other EPS, higher potency typical antipsychotics are generally more likely than lower potency typical agents and atypical antipsychotics to cause akathisia. Among atypical antipsychotics, comparative incidence rates between agents vary across studies; risperidone and aripiprazole may have slightly higher rates [3].

Tardive Dyskinesia

Tardive dyskinesia (TD) refers to all syndromes that occur after prolonged exposure to treatment with dopamine-blocking agents. It includes tardive dystonia and akathisia but classic TD refers to the stereotypic movements of the face, limbs, and trunk.

The majority of patients have oro-buccal-lingual dyskinesia that manifests as chewing, lip smacking, or tongue protruding movements. Symptoms are usually seen after 1–2 years of antipsychotic exposure though duration of exposure is variable. Most experts consider TD only after at least 3 months of antipsychotic exposure.

The incidence of TD varies across studies. The prevalence in patients on typical antipsychotics was 20% in a 1982 study [4]. As with other EPS, risk is highest with high-potency typical antipsychotics. But the risk with atypical agents appears to be higher than previously reported. A recent review reports annual rates as 5.5% for typical antipsychotics and 3.9% for atypical antipsychotics [5]. Risk is likely to be lower if lower potency typical antipsychotics or atypical antipsychotics are used. Among atypical agents, risperidone is the most likely and clozapine and quetiapine are least likely to cause TD [2].

Proposed risk factors for developing TD are older age, female gender, African-American race, history of other extrapyramidal symptoms, or other neurologic dysfunction. None have been consistently proven. Dose is not clearly correlated with TD prevalence though antipsychotic treatment with the lowest possible dose for a short duration is generally recommended. Though TD risk does increase with length of treatment, duration of antipsychotic exposure alone does not explain the differences in prevalence and severity of TD resulting from antipsychotic treatment across studies.

The course of TD is difficult to determine. TD can spontaneously resolve, especially in younger patients [6]. Stopping the medication resolves TD in some but not all patients. In the immediate period after stopping the antipsychotic, there may be a withdrawal dyskinesia and so patients have to be observed over a period of at least weeks to months to determine if TD has resolved.

> ***Risk of EPS is highest with high-potency typical antipsychotics; low-potency typical antipsychotics and atypical antipsychotics are equivalent in their risk.***

Clinical Features

Acute dystonia affects the head and neck commonly. Examples are oculogyric crisis (bilateral elevation of visual gaze due to ocular muscle spasm), laryngeal dystonia (speech difficulties due to laryngeal spasm), blepharospasm (sustained involuntary closing of eyelids), trismus (spasm of the masticatory muscles or lockjaw), and torticollis (asymmetric neck position). Tardive dystonia is also focal in onset and starts in the face and neck regions but can unfortunately spread to other body parts.

Akathisia is a sensation of motor restlessness that is present in the entire body. Patients experiencing it are extremely uncomfortable and pace to relieve the discomfort.

TD often presents as involuntary, stereotypical movements of the mouth such as lip smacking, chewing, and tongue protrusions. It also manifests as facial grimacing, eyebrow furrowing, eye closing, and rapid movements of fingers and toes. If it affects the larynx, it can result in speech or respiratory difficulties. In clinical practice, TD is often not distressing to patients even when significant to observers.

> ***Dystonia and TD more commonly affect face, neck, and upper trunk.***

Diagnosis

An abnormal involuntary movements (AIMS) scale is used to screen for EPS and provide quantitative assessment. Antipsychotic-induced movement disorders are diagnosed solely on clinical examination and history of antipsychotic exposure. No additional testing is needed or useful. In patients with additional neurologic signs or symptoms, testing may be necessary to rule out nonmedication etiologies or serious medication-related complications like serotonin syndrome and neuroleptic malignant syndrome.

> ***Diagnosis is clinical; any lab testing is only to rule out serious complications like neuroleptic malignant syndrome or serotonin syndrome.***

Management

Movement disorders can occasionally be seen with psychiatric illnesses like schizophrenia, obsessive compulsive disorder, and Tourette syndrome, in the absence of medications. Other conditions to be considered in the differential for movement disorders are central nervous system infections, metabolic disorders, neurodegenerative disease, and seizure disorder. Restless legs syndrome should be considered in the differential of a patient with akathisia.

Specific treatment strategies for each disorder are summarized as follows.

Dystonia

Anticholinergic medications can be prophylactically used in the initial week of antipsychotic treatment to reduce the risk of acute dystonia. It is common in clinical practice to continue anticholinergic agents for long-term prophylaxis but there is no evidence to support this.

If a patient develops acute severe dystonia on an antipsychotic, parenteral anticholinergic treatment with benztropine or diphenhydramine should be administered immediately. Patient should be monitored for laryngeal involvement, which can be life threatening. Usually, dystonia responds to a single dose but treatment can be repeated if necessary. In milder cases of dystonia, oral anticholinergics are sufficient for immediate treatment. Most clinicians treat with oral anticholinergic agents for a few days after an acute event to prevent relapse. It is also recommended to change the antipsychotic to an agent with lesser propensity to cause dystonia. If mild subjective muscle stiffness occurs without frank dystonia, the antipsychotic can be continued if necessary. The decision to continue the offending antipsychotic is based on severity of the dystonia, long-term effects of anticholinergic use, and the clinical need for the offending antipsychotic. If medication is switched, an agent with lesser risk for dystonia should be used.

Anticholinergics can be used for tardive dystonia also but response is not as robust. Other agents that can be tried are benzodiazepines, muscle relaxants, levodopa, and botulinum toxin injection [2]. The offending agent should be discontinued. Poor treatment response may be due to coexisting parkinsonism and also because dystonias can occur with advancing age even without dopamine-blocking medications.

In any patient with dystonia, a diagnosis of neuroleptic malignant syndrome should be considered especially if other systemic features are present.

Anticholinergic medications treat acute dystonia but there is little evidence to support using them for long-term prophylaxis.

Akathisia

There is no good evidence for medications in preventing akathisia. When it occurs, patients should be assessed for symptoms of parkinsonism. For treatment of akathisia, reducing the dose of antipsychotic may help. If this strategy is ineffective, pharmacological options exist. Propranolol is considered first-line treatment. Selective beta-blockers without central nervous system activity such as atenolol or metoprolol are not effective. Propranolol has the potential to worsen bradycardia, hypotension, asthma, heart block but the small doses used for treating EPS are generally well tolerated. Benzodiazepines are often used though evidence is limited. Anticholinergic agents and antihistamines are also often used in clinical practice. Other agents that have been tried are mirtazapine, clonidine, trazodone, and amantadine. If none of these are effective, it may be necessary to switch the agent to one that is less likely to cause akathisia. Restlessness and agitation from the underlying illness should be considered as a cause before changing the antipsychotic. If the akathisia is medication induced, it resolves with stopping the antipsychotic.

Propranolol is first-line treatment for akathisia; anticholinergic medications and benzodiazepines are less effective.

Tardive Dyskinesia

There is no evidence for any medication in preventing TD. The only prevention is choosing an antipsychotic that has lesser propensity to cause TD.

TD may resolve spontaneously, especially in younger people. But besides age, there are no factors to determine the likelihood of TD persistence. If TD is mild and not bothersome to the patient, it can be left untreated. If the symptom is impairing, antipsychotic discontinuation should be considered. If the antipsychotic is continued, pharmacological agents can be tried though efficacy is limited. Anticholinergic medications are not very helpful and may even worsen TD, especially in elderly patients. However, TD cannot be reliably distinguished from other EPS and anticholinergic agents may be effective by treating other symptoms. In clinical practice, agents that are tried include anticholinergics, benzodiazepines, amantadine, levetiracetam, and beta-blockers. All have shown only minimal efficacy. Tetrabenazine, a dopamine-depleting agent, has shown the best efficacy in treating TD but has many side effects and is rarely used for this indication [2]. Some clinicians try Vitamin E as it is well tolerated though efficacy is limited. If antipsychotic is changed, an agent with lesser risk for TD should be selected.

Stopping the antipsychotic may paradoxically worsen the TD and increasing the dose has actually been suggested as a strategy in refractory cases. However, unless the TD is significantly impairing, this is not recommended since long-term course of this strategy is not known. A more effective strategy might be to change medication to clozapine or quetiapine as this may reduce TD.

> *Anticholinergic medications are widely used to treat TD but efficacy is limited; course of TD is variable and stopping medication may not reverse symptoms.*

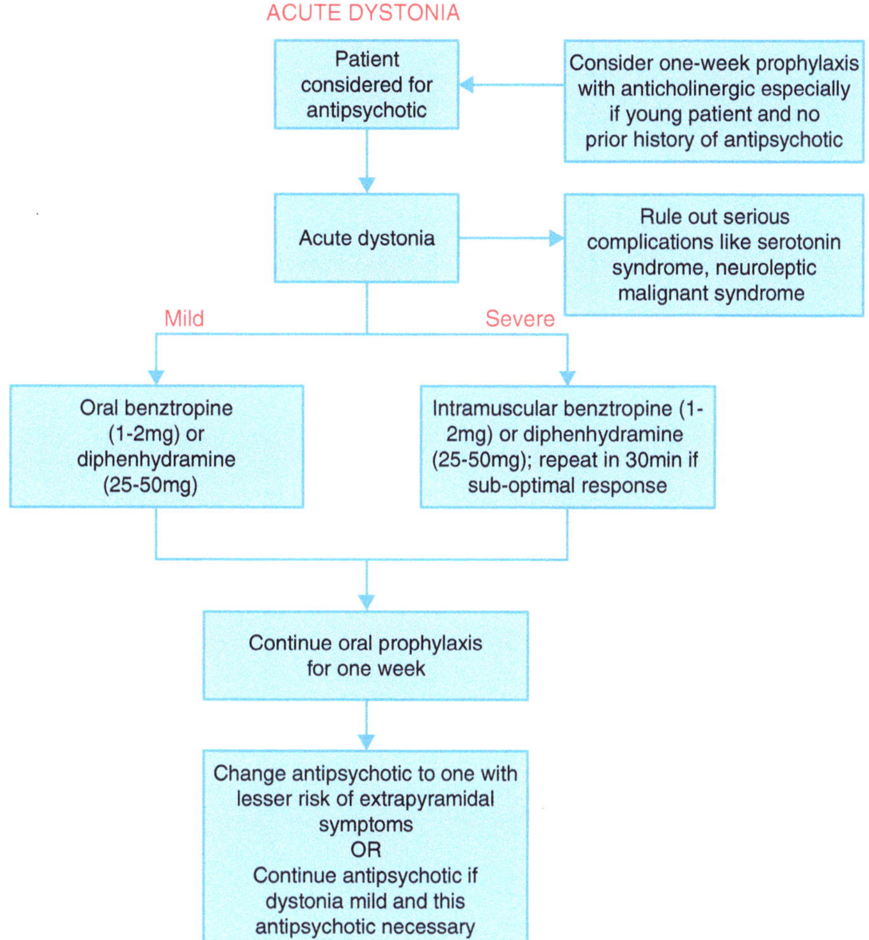

ACUTE DYSTONIA
Patient considered for antipsychotic
Consider one-week prophylaxis with anticholinergic especially if young patient and no prior history of antipsychotic
Acute dystonia
Rule out serious complications like serotonin syndrome, neuroleptic malignant syndrome
Mild
Severe
Oral benztropine (1-2mg) or diphenhydramine (25-50mg)
Intramuscular benztropine (1-2mg) or diphenhydramine (25-50mg); repeat in 30min if sub-optimal response
Continue oral prophylaxis for one week
Change antipsychotic to one with lesser risk of extrapyramidal symptoms
OR
Continue antipsychotic if dystonia mild and this antipsychotic necessary

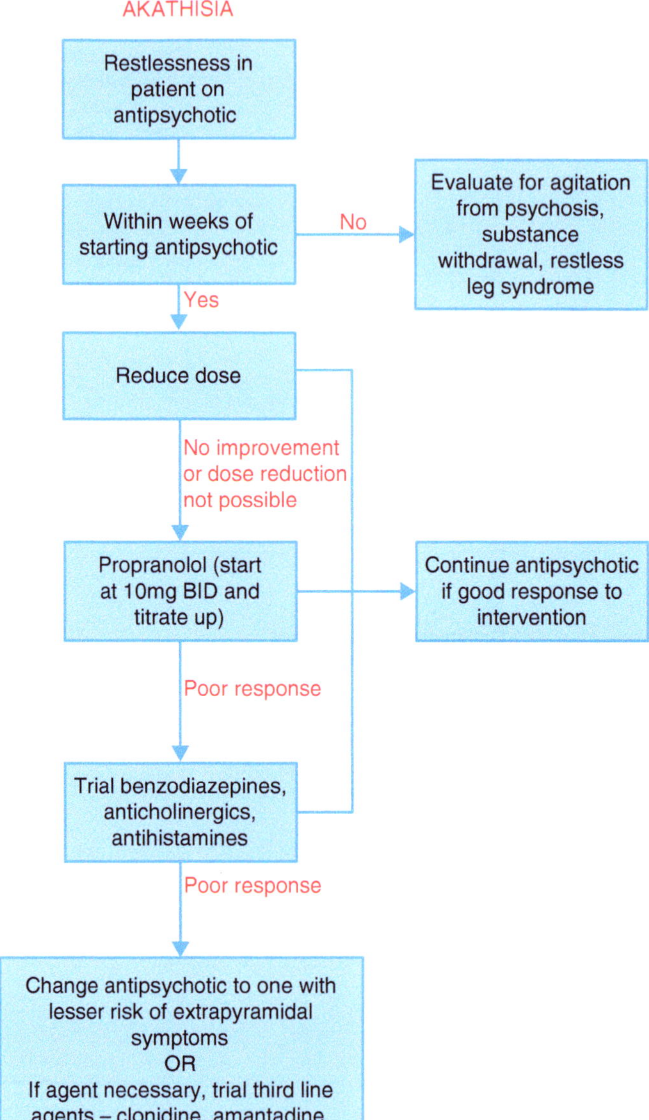
AKATHISIA
Restlessness in patient on antipsychotic
Within weeks of starting antipsychotic
No
Evaluate for agitation from psychosis, substance withdrawal, restless leg syndrome
Yes
Reduce dose
No improvement or dose reduction not possible
Propranolol (start at 10mg BID and titrate up)
Continue antipsychotic if good response to intervention
Poor response
Trial benzodiazepines, anticholinergics, antihistamines
Poor response
Change antipsychotic to one with lesser risk of extrapyramidal symptoms
OR
If agent necessary, trial third line agents – clonidine, amantadine, mirtazapine, trazodone

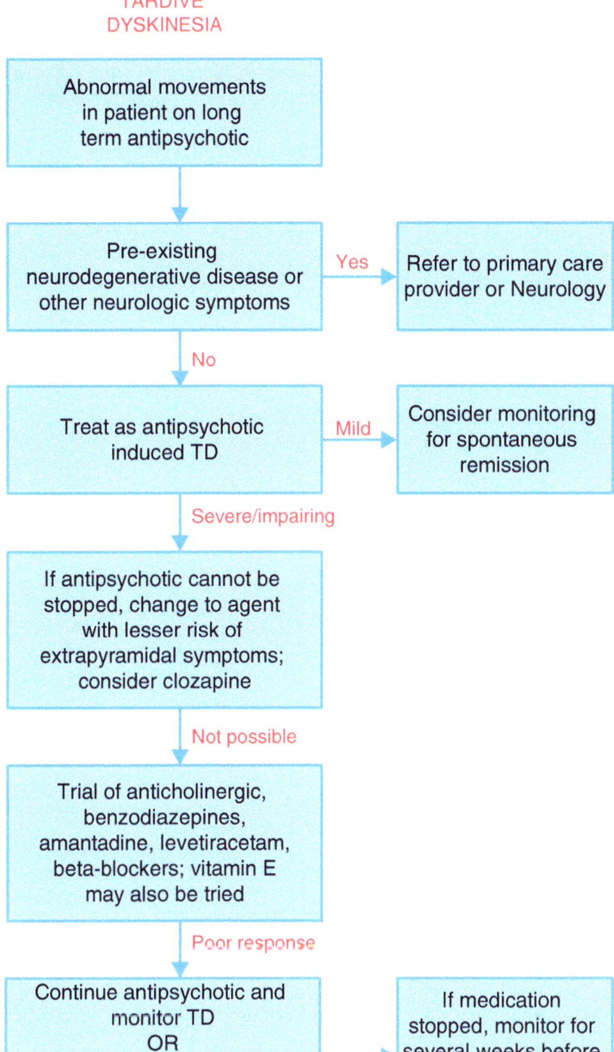

TARDIVE DYSKINESIA
Abnormal movements in patient on long term antipsychotic
Pre-existing neurodegenerative disease or other neurologic symptoms
Yes
Refer to primary care provider or Neurology
No
Treat as antipsychotic induced TD
Mild
Consider monitoring for spontaneous remission
Severe/impairing
If antipsychotic cannot be stopped, change to agent with lesser risk of extrapyramidal symptoms; consider clozapine
Not possible
Trial of anticholinergic, benzodiazepines, amantadine, levetiracetam, beta-blockers; vitamin E may also be tried
Poor response
Continue antipsychotic and monitor TD
OR
Consider tetrabenazine in conjunction with neurology if severe TD
If medication stopped, monitor for several weeks before assessing for TD resolution

References

1. Leucht S, Cipriani A, Spineli L, Mavridis D, Orey D, Richter F, et al. Comparative efficacy and tolerability of 15 antipsychotic drugs in schizophrenia: a multiple-treatments meta-analysis. Lancet. 2013;382(9896):951–62.
2. Dayalu P, Chou KL. Antipsychotic-induced extrapyramidal symptoms and their management. Expert Opin Pharmacother. 2008;9(9):1451–62.
3. Kane JM, Fleischhacker WW, Hansen L, Perlis R, Pikalov III A, Assuncao-Talbott S. Akathisia: an updated review focusing on second-generation antipsychotics. J Clin Psychiatry. 2009;70(5):627–43.
4. Kane JM, Smith JM. Tardive dyskinesia: prevalence and risk factors, 1959 to 1979. Arch Gen Psychiatry. 1982;39(4):473–81.
5. Correll CU, Schenk EM. Tardive dyskinesia and new antipsychotics. Curr Opin Psychiatry. 2008;21(2):151–6.
6. Smith JM, Baldessarini RJ. Changes in prevalence, severity, and recovery in tardive dyskinesia with age. Arch Gen Psychiatry. 1980;37(12):1368–73.

Chapter 38
Tics

Tics are hyperkinetic movements that are repetitive, rapid, nonrhythmic, and may include vocalizations.

Pathology

Tics result from disruptions in the connection between the basal ganglia and its connections to the thalamus and cortex. Disruptions of gamma aminobutyric acid (GABA) as well as serotonin and histamine transmission are implicated.

Etiology

Tics are often transient and benign. Cocaine and other stimulant use can cause tics. Neurodegenerative disorders can cause tics. Tourette syndrome, a childhood neurobehavioral disorder, is diagnosed when there are persistent motor and vocal tics.

Psychotropic Medications and Tics

Tics are seen in children treated with stimulant medications for attention deficit hyperactivity disorder (ADHD). Available data on tics and stimulant medications are predominantly in children. Evidence is mixed on whether tics are caused/exacerbated by stimulant medications or the apparent increase is explained by higher prevalence of tics in children with ADHD [1]. Patients with ADHD do have a higher incidence of tics [2] and stimulant medications may only worsen tics at supratherapeutic doses [3]. Stopping stimulant medication reverses tics in some but not all

© Springer International Publishing AG 2017
A. Annamalai, *Medical Management of Psychotropic Side Effects*,
DOI 10.1007/978-3-319-51026-2_38

patients, indicating that these medications may only worsen or unmask rather than induce tic disorders. Rarely, Tourette syndrome is precipitated with stimulant medications in children who previously did not exhibit symptoms.

Tics may also be seen as a part of tardive dyskinesia. Occasionally, mood stabilizers exacerbate tics.

> ***Tics are commonly associated with stimulant medications; however, much of this effect may come from higher incidence of tics in children with ADHD.***

Clinical Features

Tics can present as repetitive motor activity such as blinking, grimacing, throat clearing, or as unintended vocalizations including noises and words. Tics can be suppressed only with difficulty. They do not occur during sleep.

> ***Tics are generally nonsuppressible; they do not occur during sleep.***

Diagnosis

Tic disorder is a clinical diagnosis. A thorough evaluation is warranted to rule out secondary causes such as central nervous system disorders.

> ***Lab testing for a tic disorder is necessary only to rule out secondary non-medication etiologies.***

Management

In patients with ADHD and preexisting tic disorder, nonstimulant medications like atomoxetine and second-line agents like bupropion and clonidine may be tried first. If people with tics are treated with stimulant medications, they should be monitored for worsening of tics [4]. If the tics are transient or nonimpairing, no treatment is needed. If tics develop or worsen on a stimulant medication, switching to nonstimulant medications should be considered, if possible. Persistent tics, whether or not medication related, may respond to clonidine and guanfacine. Antipsychotic medications can also be tried if tics are severe or there are other indications for this class of medications.

Nonstimulant medications may be tried as first-line medications in patients with ADHD and tics.

Clonidine and guanfacine are used for treating tics; antipsychotics should be used only for persistent symptoms or for additional indications.

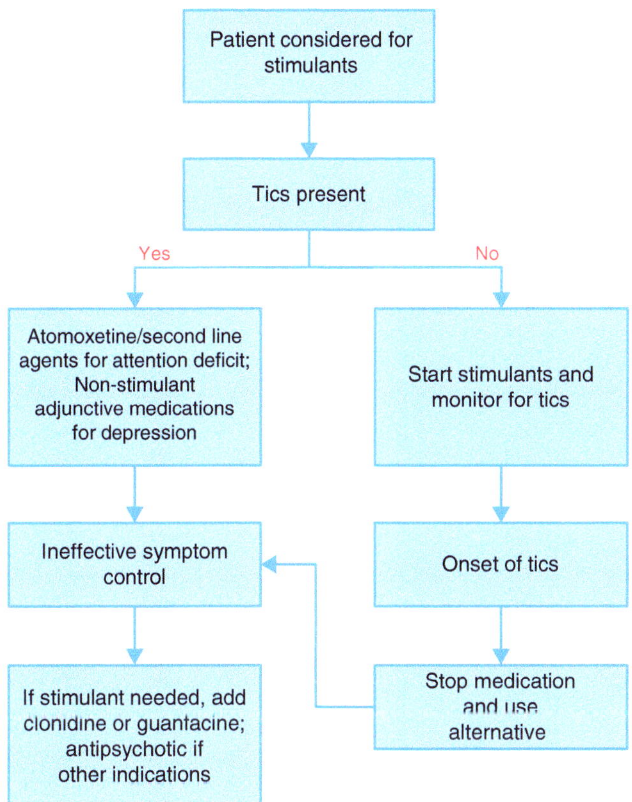

References

1. Pidsosny IC, Virani A. Pediatric psychopharmacology update: psychostimulants and tics—past, present and future. J Can Acad Child Adolesc Psychiatry. 2006;15(2):84–6.
2. Spencer TJ, Biederman J, Faraone S, Mick E, Coffey B, Geller D, et al. Impact of tic disorders on ADHD outcome across the life cycle: findings from a large group of adults with and without ADHD. Am J Psychiatry. 2001;158(4):611–7.
3. Bloch MH, Panza KE, Landeros-Weisenberger A, Leckman JF. Meta-analysis: treatment of attention-deficit/hyperactivity disorder in children with comorbid tic disorders. J Am Acad Child Adolesc Psychiatry. 2009;48(9):884–93.
4. Scahill L, Chappell PB, King RA, Leckman JF. Pharmacologic treatment of tic disorders. Child Adolesc Psychiatr Clin N Am. 2000;9(1):99–117.

Section XI
Neurologic System
Systemic Syndromes

Chapter 39
Myoclonus and Serotonin Syndrome

Myoclonus is a brief contraction of a muscle or group of muscles.

Pathology

Different neurotransmitter pathways in different regions of the brain are involved depending on the etiology.

Etiology

Myoclonus is occasionally physiologic. But it is usually seen in the presence of systemic metabolic disorders or medication toxicity. It can be seen with neurodegenerative dementing illnesses. It can occur as part of seizures. It is an important manifestation of serotonin syndrome.

Psychotropic Medications and Myoclonus

Most antidepressants and mood stabilizers can cause myoclonus with toxic overdoses. But it can occur as part of serotonin syndrome at therapeutic doses of medications. Serotonin syndrome is essentially a state of serotonin toxicity and major causes are combination of two or more serotonergic drugs and toxic ingestion of one or more serotonergic drugs. However, it can occur even with one serotonergic agent at a therapeutic dose. Adding medications that inhibit metabolism of the serotonergic agent increases the risk of serotonin syndrome due to higher serotonin levels. Almost all categories of antidepressants (selective serotonin reuptake inhibitors (SSRIs), serotonin norepinephrine reuptake inhibitors (SNRIs), tricyclic antidepressants (TCAs), monoamine oxidase inhibitors (MAOs)) carry risk of serotonin syndrome [1].

© Springer International Publishing AG 2017
A. Annamalai, *Medical Management of Psychotropic Side Effects*,
DOI 10.1007/978-3-319-51026-2_39

Serotonin syndrome can be difficult to distinguish from anticholinergic delirium and neuroleptic malignant syndrome (NMS). No symptom is pathognomonic but spontaneous clonus is highly predictive of this syndrome [2].

See table for an overview of serotonin syndrome.

Serotonin syndrome

A syndrome of excess serotonergic activity in the central and peripheral nervous system causing a range of clinical symptoms
Pathology: Increased serotonin due to stimulation of serotonin receptors (5HT1A, 5HT2 commonly implicated), increased serotonin synthesis and release in central and peripheral nervous system
Causes: Combination of serotonergic agents, initiation or dose increase of single serotonergic agents in susceptible people
Antidepressants/anxiolytics—SSRIs, SNRIs, TCAs, MAOIs, buspirone, mirtazapine
Lithium—in combination with SSRIs
Amphetamines—phentermine
Certain opiates—tramadol, fentanyl
Anti-emetics—5HT3 antagonists (e.g., ondansetron)
Anti-migraine medications—triptans
Substances of abuse—cocaine, ecstasy
Symptoms: Autonomic hyperactivity (tachycardia, hypertension, hyperthermia, flushed skin, increased intestinal activity), neuromuscular hyperactivity (muscle clonus, deep tendon hyperreflexia, hypertonia), delirium
Lab findings: No diagnostic test
Management: Supportive treatment; stopping offending agent

> ***Myoclonus is commonly seen with medication toxicity; it is also a prominent feature of serotonin syndrome.***
>
> ***Serotonin syndrome is most often caused by combination of serotonergic medications.***

Clinical Features

Myoclonus is seen as a rapid, jerky twitching of one or more muscle groups that is not suppressible. The clonus is usually in the lower extremities. In serotonin syndrome, it may be spontaneous or inducible on exam. It is commonly seen at the ankle and inducible by plantar or dorsiflexion. It is also inducible by deep tendon reflex testing. Any symptom listed in the earlier table can be seen in serotonin syndrome. Features that are more predictive of the syndrome include clonus, hyperreflexia, skin flushing, diaphoresis, agitation, hyperthermia, and hypertonicity. The latter two signs usually indicate more serious disease.

Symptoms of serotonin syndrome often occur rapidly, within hours of exposure.

Spontaneous clonus or inducible clonus along with agitation and/or autonomic disturbance is highly predictive of serotonin syndrome.

Diagnosis

Myoclonus, like any other movement abnormality, is a clinical diagnosis. As mentioned earlier, eliciting deep tendon reflexes and flexing ankle may induce clonus if it is not spontaneous.

If clonus is suspected but not evident, deep tendon reflex testing and ankle flexion should be performed to look for inducible clonus.

There are no lab tests to definitively diagnose serotonin syndrome.

Management

Myoclonus rarely occurs with psychotropic medications unless it is in the context of toxicity. Other movement abnormalities such as tics or dystonia are easily distinguishable by clinical appearance. When spontaneous clonus is seen, serotonin syndrome is a strong possibility. If there is change in mental status and/or hypertonicity, NMS should also be considered. The differentiation may depend on which particular agent was started, increased, or added prior to symptom onset.

To prevent serotonin syndrome, combination of nonpsychotropic agents with serotonergic activity should be minimized in patients on SSRIs. If patients have nonspecific symptoms, they could be monitored until either the diagnosis is clear or symptoms resolve. When serotonin syndrome is reasonably certain, prompt discontinuation of the serotonergic agent is necessary. Intensity of care depends on severity of symptoms. Usually serotonin syndrome resolves quickly with stopping the medication and provision of needed supportive care. For severe symptoms, benzodiazepines and cyproheptadine, a serotonin antagonist, may be used.

To minimize risk of recurrence, agents with lesser serotonergic activity should be used (e.g., bupropion). If the syndrome occurred due to addition of a second agent, the first medication can likely be restarted after symptoms resolve.

Prompt discontinuation of serotonergic medication is warranted if serotonin syndrome is suspected; if two serotonergic agents were used, one can still be restarted if necessary.

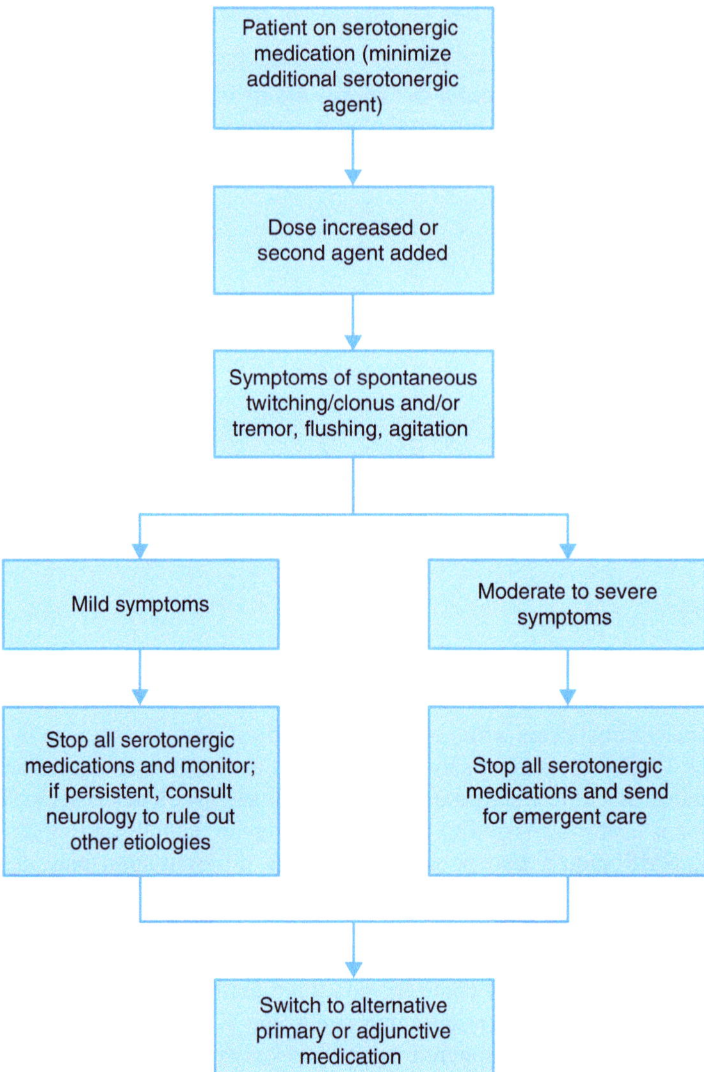

References

1. Volpi-Abadie J, Kaye AM, Kaye AD. Serotonin syndrome. Ochsner J. 2013;13(4):533–40.
2. Dunkley EJ, Isbister GK, Sibbritt D, Dawson AH, Whyte IM. The Hunter Serotonin Toxicity Criteria: simple and accurate diagnostic decision rules for serotonin toxicity. QJM. 2003;96(9):635–42.

Chapter 40
Creatine Kinase Elevation and Neuroleptic Malignant Syndrome

Creatine kinase (CK) is an enzyme released into serum in response to muscle injury. The prevalence and extent of CK elevation depends on the underlying cause.

Pathology

CK is present in many tissues. Skeletal muscle contains the majority of CK. CK has three different isoenzymes—MM, MB, BB. Ninety nine percent of skeletal muscle CK is CK-MM. Cardiac tissue has the highest concentration of CK-MB and brain tissue has high concentrations of CK-BB. Any damage to muscle causes release of CK and higher serum levels.

Etiology

CK elevation can be seen both with and without primary muscle disease. Major causes of CK elevation are listed in the table.

Creatine kinase elevation can occur due to many causes besides complications of antipsychotic use.

Causes of creatine kinase elevation

Primary neuromuscular disorders
Inflammatory myopathies (e.g., polymyositis, local myositis)
Muscular dystrophies (e.g., Duchennes)
Metabolic myopathies (e.g., inherited disorders of lipid, carbohydrate, and nucleic acid metabolism)

© Springer International Publishing AG 2017

A. Annamalai, *Medical Management of Psychotropic Side Effects*,

DOI 10.1007/978-3-319-51026-2_40

Motor neurone disease (e.g., amyotrophic lateral sclerosis—mild elevation)
Secondary or iatrogenic causes
Neuroleptic malignant syndrome (antipsychotics, antiemetics)
Malignant hyperthermia (inhalational anesthetics)
Medications (statins, fibrates, colchicine, antimalarials)
Recreational substances (cocaine, alcohol)
Acute muscle injury (trauma, seizures, surgery, intramuscular injections, infections, electrolyte imbalance)
Exercise (about threefold; peak at 24 h after exercise)
Untreated hypothyroidism (mild elevations)

Psychotropic Medications and CK Elevation

CK tends to be higher in younger people and in blacks. Values in these individuals may be a little higher than what is reported as the upper limit of normal and this should be considered when interpreting the lab value.

CK elevation is associated with antipsychotics as well as antiemetics that have dopamine-blocking properties. Neuroleptic malignant syndrome (NMS) is a rare but potentially life-threatening side effect of these medications. It is hypothesized to result from alteration of central neuroregulatory mechanisms and abnormal reaction of skeletal muscle to antipsychotics. NMS usually develops in days to weeks after exposure. See table for an overview of NMS.

Neuroleptic malignant syndrome

Neurologic syndrome with autonomic imbalance
Pathology: Unknown; possibly related to central dopamine blockade
Causes: antipsychotics, antiparkinsonian medication withdrawal, certain psychiatric conditions
Symptoms: altered mental status, muscle rigidity, hyperthermia, autonomic imbalance—usually develop in this order
Lab findings: elevated CK, elevated white cell count, multiple electrolyte abnormalities
Management: maintaining electrolyte and fluid balance, dantrolene or bromocriptine, stopping offending agent

CK is often, but not always, elevated in NMS. CK can be normal, especially in early stages. The CK is usually >1000 IU/L and sometimes as high as 100,000 IU/L. It is not a reliable marker for NMS as an isolated lab test. The incidence of NMS with antipsychotics is estimated at 0.2–3% and occurs both with typical and atypical agents [1]. While it is thought to occur more commonly with typical agents, several reports with atypical agents have been published [2].

> *Creatine kinase is often but not always elevated in neuroleptic malignant syndrome. It is one of many findings in this syndrome.*

An important but less well-known effect of antipsychotics is to elevate CK independent of the NMS syndrome. The mechanism is thought to be intermittent increase of cell membrane permeability in susceptible individuals. CK elevations more than ten times normal have been recorded in patients on antipsychotics in the absence of NMS [3]. Approximately 10% patients may have CK elevation on antipsychotics but most are asymptomatic. CK elevation is usually early in treatment but can occur even years later. It is often self-limiting. It may or may not recur if medication is stopped and rechallenged [3].

Asymptomatic creatine kinase elevation can occur in up to 10% patients on antipsychotics. It is often self-limiting and requires no intervention.

If there is significant CK elevation, it can result in rhabdomyolysis, a condition that results from injury to muscle cell membrane with potential for renal failure and other complications. See table below for an overview of rhabdomyolysis. The mean CK is higher than that in NMS. It is usually at least five times normal and can be as high as 100,000 IU/L. The exact incidence of rhabdomyolysis with antipsychotics is unknown but accounts for 10% of all rhabdomyolysis cases [4]. Higher doses and multiple antipsychotics increase risk.

Significant creatine kinase elevation can result in rhabdomyolysis, which can be seen without accompanying neuroleptic malignant syndrome.

Rhabdomyolysis

Syndrome of muscle death and release of muscle constituents into the serum and urine
Pathology: disruption of muscle cell membrane
Causes: drugs, trauma, exertion, infections
Symptoms: muscle pain or stiffness, reddish-brown urine, generalized weakness
Lab findings: elevated CK, myoglobinuria (50% cases), elevated creatinine (if renal failure has set in)
Management: maintaining electrolyte and fluid balance, stopping offending agent

Clinical Features

An elevation in CK is asymptomatic in most cases unless serious complications have set in. Occasionally, there may be mild muscle rigidity even in the absence of complications. If rhabdomyolysis or NMS has developed, the clinical picture will resemble that of these syndromes.

Mild CK elevation with antipsychotics is usually asymptomatic.

Diagnosis

There is no need to routinely test for CK in asymptomatic patients on antipsychotics. If patients complain of muscle rigidity, muscle weakness, or change in urine color, CK should be measured. There is no need to measure other markers of muscle breakdown, such as lactate dehydrogenase (LDH), aldolase, aminotransferases, as they are not as sensitive or specific as CK. If CK is approximately 1.5–2 times normal, electrolytes and creatinine should be checked.

> *There is no need to routinely test for creatine kinase in patients on antipsychotics.*

Management

If CK is elevated in a patient with severe muscular rigidity or fluctuations in vital signs or hyperthermia, patient should be evaluated immediately in the emergency room for NMS or rhabdomyolysis. In a patient with mild symptoms and no hemodynamic changes, other causes noted earlier, notably, severe exercise, alcohol, or cocaine use, should be ruled out. If CK elevation is suspected to be from antipsychotic use, it can still be continued if the elevation is mild and can be monitored. The risk of complications increases with rise in serum CK level but there is no absolute threshold at which medication should be stopped. A reasonable threshold to use for stopping the medication is if serial CK values are rising and it remains over 1000 IU/L.

Clinicians should also remember to rule out other serious psychotropic medication-related complications like serotonin syndrome, especially in the presence of altered mental status. Severe cases of serotonin syndrome can result in rhabdomyolysis and CK elevation.

If decision is made to stop medication for CK elevation, patients can be rechallenged to see if the elevation recurs. If a patient develops rhabdomyolysis, rechallenge is recommended only with a different antipsychotic. In the case of a serious complication like NMS also, rechallenge can be attempted with a different antipsychotic. Case reports exist for both successful rechallenge and recurrence of NMS with antipsychotic use [5]. The risk of NMS might be lowered by using a single agent, avoiding coadministration of lithium, selecting a lower potency antipsychotic, lower dosage medication, and waiting at least 2 weeks before rechallenge.

> *Common causes of creatine kinase elevation should be ruled out before changing the antipsychotic.*
>
> *Antipsychotic may be continued if creatine kinase elevation is <1000 IU/L and patient has no symptoms or only mild muscle stiffness.*

Rarely, rhabdomyolysis occurs with significant creatine kinase elevation in the absence of other NMS features.

After an episode of neuroleptic malignant syndrome, rechallenge with a different antipsychotic can be attempted.

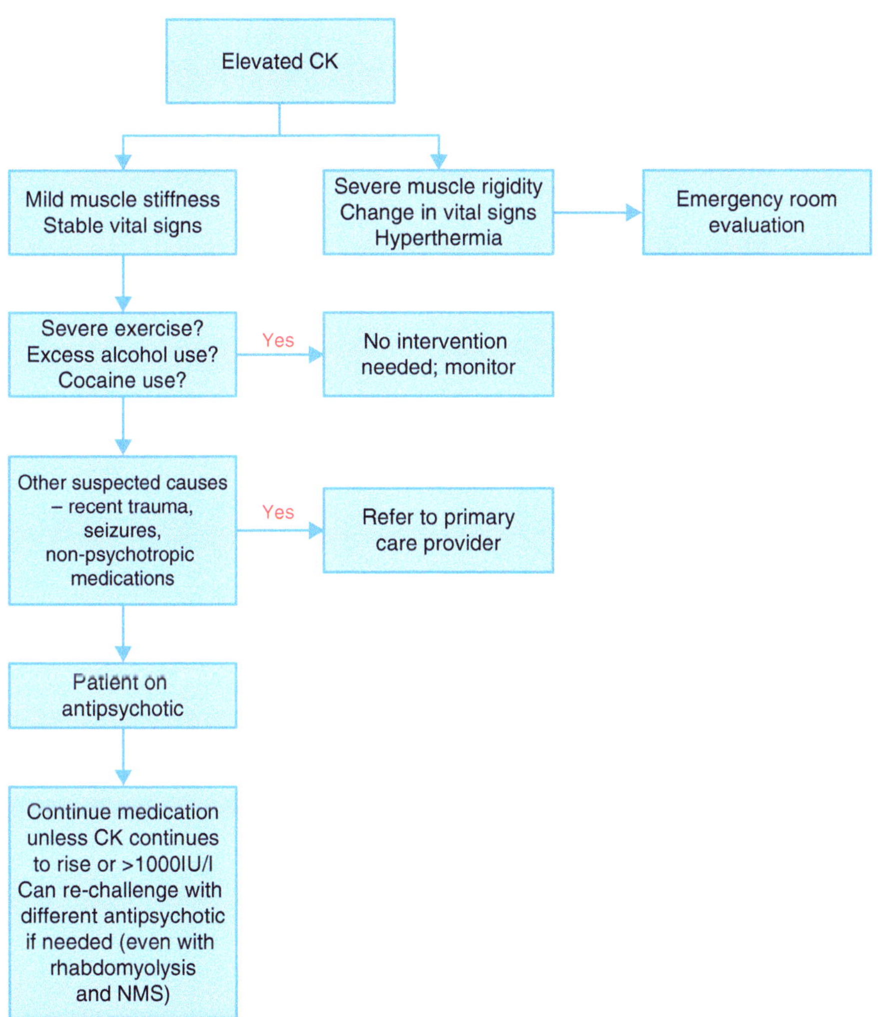

References

1. Ananth J, Parameswaran S, Gunatilake S, Burgoyne K, Sidhom T. Neuroleptic malignant syndrome and atypical antipsychotic drugs. The Journal of clinical psychiatry. 2004;65(4): 464–70.
2. Berman BD. Neuroleptic malignant syndrome: a review for neurohospitalists. Neurohospitalist. 2011;1(1):41–7.
3. Meltzer HY, Cola PA, Parsa M. Marked elevations of serum creatine kinase activity associated with antipsychotic drug treatment. Neuropsychopharmacology. 1996;15(4):395–405.
4. Packard K, Price P, Hanson A. Antipsychotic use and the risk of rhabdomyolysis. J Pharm Pract. 2014;27(5):501–12.
5. Wells AJ, Sommi RW, Crismon ML. Neuroleptic rechallenge after neuroleptic malignant syndrome: case report and literature review. Drug Intell Clin Pharm. 1988;22(6):475–80.

Section XII
Neurologic System
Other Conditions

Chapter 41
Seizures

Seizure is a sudden onset of behavior change due to a brain dysfunction. It occurs due to excessive, hypersynchronous discharge from cerebral cortical neurons. Epilepsy is a disorder characterized by recurrent unprovoked seizures.

Pathology

The potential mechanisms by which medications affect the seizure threshold are neurotransmitter changes (e.g., dopamine blockade, gaba aminobutyric acid (GABA) inhibition, alpha adrenoceptor down-regulation), cerebral neuronal effects (e.g., chloride influx inhibition), cerebral cortex irritation, and changes in cerebral blood flow.

Etiology

Seizures can be caused by acute neurologic dysfunction or temporary metabolic abnormalities. Medications are a cause of provoked seizures. Opioid analgesics, some penicillin derivative antibiotics, and antineoplastic agents are examples of medications other than psychotropics that can provoke seizures. In many patients with epilepsy, a cause cannot be identified and is presumed to be a genetic predisposition.

© Springer International Publishing AG 2017

A. Annamalai, *Medical Management of Psychotropic Side Effects*,

DOI 10.1007/978-3-319-51026-2_41

Psychotropic Medications and Seizures

The relationship between psychotropic medications and seizures is complicated. Psychiatric disease is more frequent among people with epilepsy. Effects of individual medications on seizure threshold vary but generally psychotropic drugs reduce seizure threshold.

Patient factors predisposing to increased risk of seizures with offending medications are shown in the table.

Risk factors for medication-induced seizures

Previous history of seizures
Family history of epilepsy
Central nervous system disorders (e.g., stroke, HIV encephalopathy, head injury)
Extremes of age
Renal and hepatic dysfunction
Polypharmacy
Concomitant substance use and withdrawal

The seizure incidence rates with antidepressants and antipsychotics range from 0.1 to 1.5% at therapeutic doses. This is slightly higher than the 0.07–0.09% incidence of first unprovoked seizure in the general population [1]. In overdose situations, the risk increases significantly.

Medication-induced seizures are dose related. They usually occur within several weeks of medication initiation or dosage increase.

> *At therapeutic doses, the risk of seizure with psychotropic medications is only slightly increased.*

Almost all antipsychotics decrease the seizure threshold. Lower potency agents may be generally higher risk than high potency agents. But there are individual variations between agents. Chlorpromazine and clozapine carry the highest risk among typical and atypical agents, respectively [2]. There may be an increased risk overall with atypical versus typical agents [3].

As with all agents, risk with clozapine increases with dose and is about 4% over 600 mg/day. The serum level is a more accurate predictor of seizure risk and levels >1300 ng/mL carry a substantial risk of seizures [4].

> *Risk of seizures with clozapine increases with dose and is significantly higher over 600 mg/day.*

Among antidepressants, tricyclic antidepressants (TCAs) decrease seizure threshold and increase seizure risk [5]. The risk with selective serotonin reuptake inhibitors (SSRIs) is considered to be no higher than in the general population. Bupropion, a dopamine and norepinephrine reuptake inhibitor, increases seizure risk slightly with a rate of 0.36% [6] at doses over 300 mg/day; risk is comparable to tricyclic antidepressants. Risk with bupropion can be minimized by using sustained or extended release formulations and lowest effective doses. Monoamine oxidase inhibitors do not appear to increase seizure risk at therapeutic doses.

Risk of seizure with bupropion is small if doses <300 mg/day and sustained/ extended release formulations are used.

Many mood stabilizers are also antiepileptic agents. There are case reports of seizures with lithium at therapeutic doses but the risk is small and mainly in people with predisposition to seizures.

Stimulant medications have a slightly increased risk of 0.6% in children treated for attention deficit disorder. The risk is higher if there is an underlying predisposition to seizures [7] though they can be used safely in patients with well-controlled epilepsy. Benzodiazepine withdrawal can precipitate seizures.

Cocaine and other stimulant intoxication and alcohol withdrawal are nonprescription substances that can provoke seizures.

Psychotropic medications and seizure risk

Category	Higher risk	Lower risk
Antipsychotics	Clozapine, chlorpromazine	Olanzapine, risperidone, quetiapine, ziprasidone, aripiprazole, haloperidol, fluphenazine, trifluoperazine
Antidepressants	TCAs (Clomipramine, amitriptyline, imipramine, nortriptyline, desipramine), maprotiline	SSRIs (Fluoxetine, citalopram, sertraline, fluvoxamine, paroxetine), venlafaxine, trazodone, tranylcypromine, phenelzine
	Bupropion	
Mood stabilizers	None	Lithium
Stimulants	None	Both amphetamine and methylphenidate categories

Clinical Features

Seizure is characterized by partial or complete lack of awareness of surroundings and abnormal motor activity. When the motor activity is focal with partial loss of awareness, the seizure is classified as complex partial. Generalized motor activity with loss of consciousness is termed tonic–clinic seizure. When there is loss of consciousness with sudden absence of activity, seizures are termed absence seizures. Complex partial and generalized tonic–clonic seizures are usually accompanied by motor, sensory, or autonomic aura.

Medication-induced seizures are more likely to be generalized and tonic–clonic.

Psychogenic seizures are another possibility. Patients usually do not exhibit symptoms of tongue biting, urinary incontinence, self-injury; eyes are more likely to be closed; often do not have total loss of consciousness; and episode lasts longer.

> ***Medication-induced seizures are usually generalized tonic–clonic seizures.***

Diagnosis

An epileptiform seizure should be differentiated from a complex migraine, transient ischemic attack, vasovagal episodes, syncope, panic attacks, sleep disorders, and movement disorders. A new onset seizure has to be differentiated from psychogenic seizures. However, clinical observation alone often cannot reliably distinguish between psychogenic and epileptiform seizures.

For a new onset epileptiform seizure, it is important to assess for underlying reversible etiologies. This requires further lab testing or imaging as warranted by the clinical situation. Epileptiform seizures have to be confirmed by electroencephalography (EEG) or video EEG monitoring.

> ***Etiologies besides medications should be considered with a new onset seizure.***

Management

When starting patients on psychotropic medications, if there are any risk factors for seizures, medications with lesser risk should be used wherever possible. Low starting doses, slow dose titration, and maintaining minimally effective medication doses are effective strategies to reduce the risk of drug-induced seizures. If a patient does develop seizures while on a psychotropic medication, other causes should be ruled out. If the seizure developed in the time period following a new medication or dose increase and no other cause is identified, the offending medication should be reduced or stopped. In suspected medication-induced seizure, it is not necessary to obtain an EEG but either an EEG or a neurology referral should be considered if primary epilepsy is a possibility.

Clozapine is a special case where switching medication may not be possible. If dose reduction and eliminating other risk factors is not possible, an anticonvulsant may be added. Valproate is effective for generalized seizures and is often used as it does not affect clozapine serum levels and additive risk of neutropenia is small. Many experts recommend adding valproate prophylactically at clozapine doses >600 mg/day and serum levels >800 ng/mL though higher thresholds have also been proposed [4]. Dosing of valproate for seizures is similar to doses used for mood disturbance. Even with concomitant valproate, goal should be to keep clozapine dose as low as clinically possible. Many factors affect clozapine serum levels, such as cigarette smoke, and this should be considered when monitoring clozapine levels.

> ***Slow dose titration and maintaining lowest effective doses are key strategies to prevent medication-induced seizures; medication may need to be switched if seizure occurs.***
>
> ***Anticonvulsants can be considered for prophylaxis with clozapine at doses >600 mg/day and serum levels >800 ng/mL.***
>
> ***Valproate is usually chosen for prophylaxis and treatment of clozapine-induced seizures as it does not affect clozapine serum levels and is low risk for additive neutropenia.***

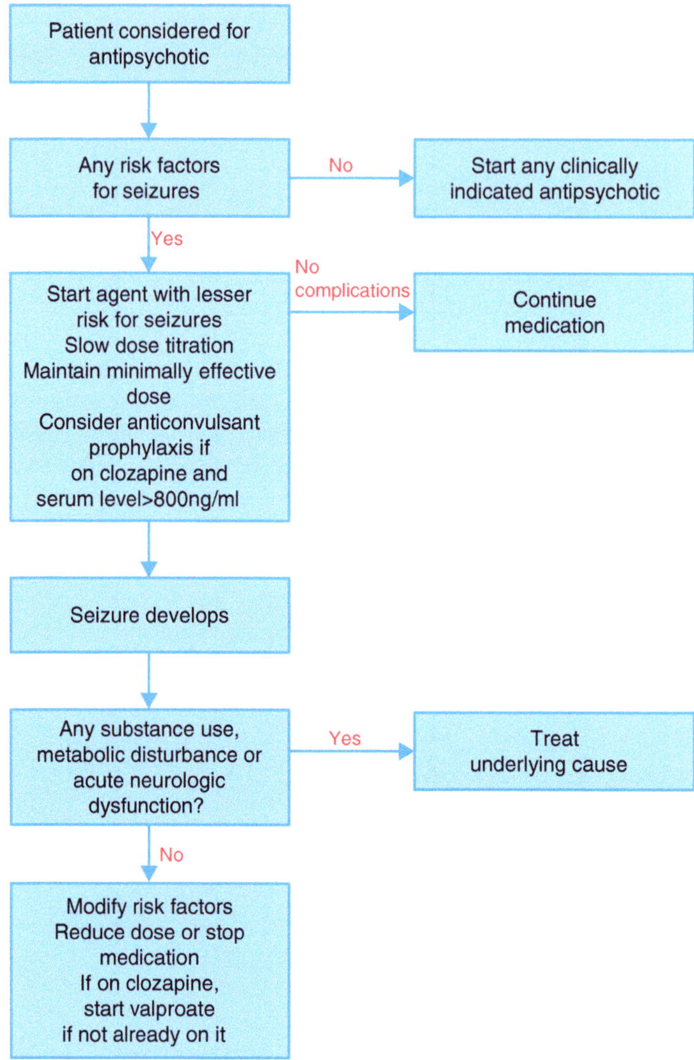

References

1. Pisani F, Oteri G, Costa C, Di Raimondo G, Di Perri R. Effects of psychotropic drugs on seizure threshold. Drug Saf. 2002;25(2):91–110.
2. Hedges D, Jeppson K, Whitehead P. Antipsychotic medication and seizures: a review. Drugs Today (Barc). 2003;39(7):551–7.
3. Lertxundi U, Hernandez R, Medrano J, Domingo-Echaburu S, Garcia M, Aguirre C. Antipsychotics and seizures: higher risk with atypicals? Seizure. 2013;22(2):141–3.

4. Caetano D. Use of anticonvulsants as prophylaxis for seizures in patients on clozapine. Australas Psychiatry. 2014;22(1):78–83.
5. Rosenstein DL, Nelson JC, Jacobs SC. Seizures associated with antidepressants: a review. J Clin Psychiatry. 1993;54(8):289–99.
6. Johnston JA, Lineberry CG, Ascher JA, Davidson J, Khayrallah MA, Feighner JP, et al. A 102-center prospective study of seizure in association with bupropion. J Clin Psychiatry. 1991;52(11):450–6.
7. Hemmer SA, Pasternak JF, Zecker SG, Trommer BL. Stimulant therapy and seizure risk in children with ADHD. Pediatr Neurol. 2001;24(2):99–102.

Chapter 42
Altered Mental Status

An acute confusional state or delirium is characterized by a disturbance in attention and memory that develops over a short period of time. It is usually encountered in a hospital setting, where it is seen in as much as 50% elderly people with multiple medical comorbidities. But it can also be detected in an outpatient setting and in these cases, psychotropic medications should be considered as a possible etiology.

Pathology

Acute change in mental status or delirium is multifactorial in origin. It involves both cortical and subcortical mechanisms; acetylcholine is a key neurotransmitter in its pathogenesis. Many factors increase underlying vulnerability—older age, dementia, Parkinson disease, past stroke. Many conditions act as precipitating factors—volume depletion, systemic infections, polypharmacy.

Etiology

A delirious state is caused by an underlying medical condition, medication side effect, or substance intoxication or withdrawal. Most common etiologies, especially those likely to be encountered in an outpatient setting are listed in the following table.

© Springer International Publishing AG 2017

A. Annamalai, *Medical Management of Psychotropic Side Effects*,

DOI 10.1007/978-3-319-51026-2_42

Major etiologies of delirium

Medications—opioids, sedatives, antihistamines, muscle relaxants, steroids, anticonvulsants, psychotropic medications
Substances—acute ingestion of any substance, ethanol or benzodiazepine withdrawal
Central nervous system disorders—acute sequelae of fall, nonconvulsive seizure, onset of stroke
Systemic illnesses—acute urinary or respiratory tract infection, hypertensive emergency, acute hyperglycemia, hyperammonemia from liver failure, acute hypoxemia or hypercarbia from exacerbation of lung disease, electrolyte disturbance from dehydration/acute renal failure

Psychotropic Medications and Delirium

Most cognitive impairments associated with psychotropic medications are chronic (see Appendix). Delirium is a rare side effect of psychotropic agents in the absence of toxicity. Medications associated with delirium generally have significant anticholinergic activity. Polypharmacy with multiple medications with anticholinergic or sedating properties increases the risk of delirium.

Antipsychotics associated with higher anticholinergic properties include clozapine, olanzapine, and some medications in the phenothiazine class of typical antipsychotics. Quetiapine also has some anticholinergic properties [1]. A risk factor that significantly increases chances of delirium with clozapine is combination with other anticholinergic medications [2]. Combining with benzodiazepines also increases risk [3]. Clozapine withdrawal also may cause delirium, likely from cholinergic rebound [4].

Tricyclic antidepressants also can cause delirium at therapeutic doses and the effect is related to serum level of the medication [5]. Selective serotonergic reuptake inhibitors may cause delirium via hyponatremia or the life-threatening complication of serotonin syndrome. Acute withdrawal from benzodiazepines is a well-known cause of delirium. Many antihistamines have potent anticholinergic activity and can exacerbate delirium. Diphenhydramine is a notable example. Hydroxyzine is less anticholinergic. Delirium associated with electroconvulsive therapy may be exacerbated with concurrent use of some medications, notably clozapine and lithium. Benzodiazepines may exacerbate symptoms of delirium by causing sedation.

It is to be noted that in spite of their anticholinergic and sedating effects, quetiapine, olanzapine, and benzodiazepine have some proven efficacy for treating delirium and are sometimes used for this indication.

Antipsychotics and anticholinergic side effects

Clozapine, olanzapine, low-potency typical antipsychotics	+++
Quetiapine	++
Typical antipsychotics, risperidone, ziprasidone, aripiprazole	+/−

Anticholinergic delirium is potentially life threatening. The table lists the key features.

Anticholinergic delirium

A constellation of symptoms resulting from excess anticholinergic activity in different organ systems

Pathology: Inhibition of binding of acetylcholine with muscarinic receptors in smooth muscle, ciliary muscle of the eye, secretory glands, central nervous system

Causes: Drugs (low potency antipsychotics, tricyclic antidepressants, antihistamines)

Symptoms: Delirium, dry and red skin, dry mouth, pupillary dilation, urinary retention, tachycardia, intestinal slowing

Lab findings: No diagnostic test available

Management: Supportive treatment; stopping offending agent

Delirium is not a defining feature of serotonin syndrome but agitation is commonly seen. See Chapter 39 for features of serotonin syndrome. Delirium is also seen with neuroleptic malignant syndrome (NMS), which is described in Chapter 40.

Low-potency antipsychotics, tricyclic antidepressants, some antihistamines have the potential for anticholinergic delirium; combination of agents with anticholinergic properties is a strong risk factor.

Clinical Features

Delirium, by definition, is a disturbance in awareness and attention, usually accompanied by a change in cognition. It is a deviation from the person's baseline and develops over a short period of time. It may not always be easily distinguishable from exacerbation of underlying symptoms such as thought disorganization secondary to an underlying psychotic disorder.

When psychotic symptom exacerbation is suspected, medication-induced delirium should be considered especially if agitation and disorganized thought processes are prominent.

Diagnosis

Delirium can be diagnosed clinically. Formal bedside cognitive testing can be performed [6] though not essential. Many conditions causing a change in mental status can be ruled out by a reliable history and knowledge of prior medical status. A blood glucose level should be determined to rule out acute hyperglycemia. Urine toxicology, infectious disease workup, serum electrolytes, and appropriate imaging may be necessary depending on the suspected underlying condition.

If change in mental status is mild and there are no other accompanying symptoms or change in vital signs, stopping the medication will serve as a diagnostic test.

Delirium is a clinical diagnosis; lab tests are to rule out underlying medical conditions.

Management

If any patient presents with altered mental status, first step should be to determine if delirium is the cause rather than underlying psychiatric symptomatology. If acute and significantly different from baseline, generally they should be referred for an urgent evaluation to rule out a life-threatening illness. This includes medical conditions and psychotropic adverse effects like serotonin syndrome. An outpatient assessment may be considered if the mental status change is not a definitive change from baseline, no other symptoms are present, vital signs are stable, and resources for outpatient workup are accessible.

The medication list should be reviewed to look for offending medications. If a nonpsychotropic medication is suspected, patient should be referred to the appropriate prescriber. If a psychotropic medication was newly started, dose can be lowered. If needed, it can be stopped as a trial. If patient is on more than one offending agent, the medication that is less critical may be stopped first. If delirium reverses after stopping the psychotropic agent, the same medication should preferably not be restarted and maintained at the same dose.

If serotonin syndrome or NMS are suspected at any stage, the potential offending medication should be immediately stopped. If these syndromes are suspected, then the medication should not be restarted. If delirium occurred on a combination of medications, the medication that is clinically necessary may be cautiously restarted. See Chapters 39 and 40 for further discussion of serotonin syndrome and NMS.

Mild changes in cognitive status without systemic symptoms can be assessed as outpatient.

If psychotropic-induced delirium is suspected, dose reduction can be trialed before stopping the medication.

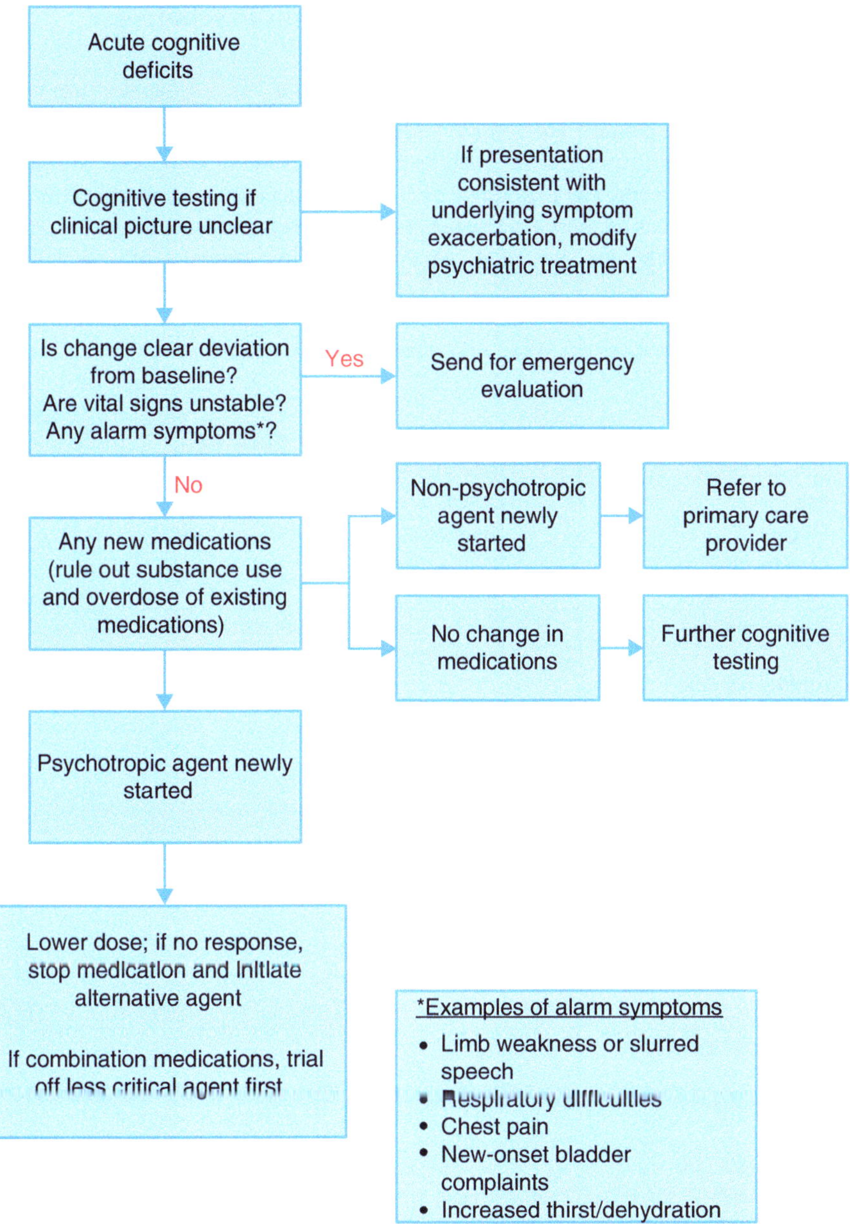
Acute cognitive deficits
Cognitive testing if clinical picture unclear
If presentation consistent with underlying symptom exacerbation, modify psychiatric treatment
Is change clear deviation from baseline?
Are vital signs unstable?
Any alarm symptoms*?
Yes
Send for emergency evaluation
No
Any new medications (rule out substance use and overdose of existing medications)
Non-psychotropic agent newly started
Refer to primary care provider
No change in medications
Further cognitive testing
Psychotropic agent newly started
Lower dose; if no response, stop medication and initiate alternative agent

If combination medications, trial off less critical agent first
*Examples of alarm symptoms
• Limb weakness or slurred speech
• Respiratory difficulties
• Chest pain
• New-onset bladder complaints
• Increased thirst/dehydration

Appendix: Chronic Cognitive Deficits from Psychotropic Medications

Many cognitive deficits are reported secondary to mood stabilizers and other psychotropic medications. Topiramate is a notable example associated with global cognitive impairment. The magnitude of cognitive effect with psychotropic medications is uncertain as patients already may have underlying deficits due to psychiatric illness. See table for potential adverse cognitive effects of psychotropic medications.

Psychotropic medications associated with cognitive impairment [7]

Mood stabilizers [8]	
Topiramate	Impaired global cognitive function
Carbamazepine	Decreased learning, visuospatial processing
Valproate	Deficits in attention, memory
Lithium	Diminished verbal memory, creativity
Lamotrigine	Minimal to none
Oxcarbazepine	Minimal to none
Antipsychotics	Possible impairment in attention, memory, visuospatial function, processing speed, planning
Antidepressants	
SSRIs[a]	None
SNRIs[b]	None
TCAs[c]	Decreased verbal learning, memory
Benzodiazepines	Impaired attention, arousal, memory, reaction time
Anticholinergics	Cognitive dulling, gross impairment in attention

[a]Selective serotonin reuptake inhibitors
[b]Serotonin norepinephrine reuptake inhibitors
[c]Tricyclic antidepressants

References

1. Chew ML, Mulsant BH, Pollock BG, Lehman ME, Greenspan A, Kirshner MA, et al. A model of anticholinergic activity of atypical antipsychotic medications. Schizophr Res. 2006;88(1–3):63–72.
2. Centorrino F, Albert MJ, Drago-Ferrante G, Koukopoulos AE, Berry JM, Baldessarini RJ. Delirium during clozapine treatment: incidence and associated risk factors. Pharmacopsychiatry. 2003;36(4):156–60.
3. Jackson CW, Markowitz JS, Brewerton TD. Delirium associated with clozapine and benzodiazepine combinations. Ann Clin Psychiatry. 1995;7(3):139–41.
4. Stanilla JK, de Leon J, Simpson GM. Clozapine withdrawal resulting in delirium with psychosis: a report of three cases. J Clin Psychiatry. 1997;58(6):252–5.

5. Livingston RL, Zucker DK, Isenberg K, Wetzel RD. Tricyclic antidepressants and delirium. J Clin Psychiatry. 1983;44(5):173–6.
6. Wong CL, Holroyd-Leduc J, Simel DL, Straus SE. Does this patient have delirium? Value of bedside instruments. JAMA. 2010;304(7):779–86.
7. Goldberg J. Adverse cognitive effects of psychotropic medications. In: Goldberg JF, Burdick K, editors. Cognitive dysfunction in bipolar disorder. 1st ed. Washington, DC: American Psychiatric Publishing, Inc.; 2008. p. 137–58.
8. Gualtieri CT, Johnson LG. Comparative neurocognitive effects of 5 psychotropic anticonvulsants and lithium. MedGenMed. 2006;8(3):46.

Section XIII
Miscellaneous

Chapter 43
Xerostomia

Xerostomia, a feeling of dry mouth, is often caused by medications. Common non-psychotropic causes are other medications (e.g., decongestants, diuretics), substance use (e.g., tobacco, methamphetamine), and excessive mouth breathing (as in nasal congestion). Less common causes are chemotherapy, radiation therapy, and Sjogren's syndrome. In addition to oral discomfort, a complication of dry mouth is dental caries.

Psychotropic Medications and Xerostomia

Any psychotropic medication with anticholinergic effects can reduce salivary secretions and cause dry mouth. Low-potency typical antipsychotics, olanzapine, and clozapine are potential offenders.

Other additive causes including poor water intake, volume depletion, high salt intake, and elevated blood sugar should be addressed. Sipping sugarless fluids, chewing sugarless gum, or using a glycerin-based oral saliva substitute can be tried for symptom relief [1]. Pilocarpine, a cholinomimetic, is used in some conditions but it generally has no role in medication-induced xerostomia. To prevent dental caries, patients should be instructed to maintain good oral hygiene and have periodic dental visits.

Dry mouth is commonly caused by anticholinergic medications. Appropriate care should be given to prevent dental caries.

© Springer International Publishing AG 2017   281
A. Annamalai, *Medical Management of Psychotropic Side Effects*,
DOI 10.1007/978-3-319-51026-2_43

Reference

1. Mouly SJ, Orler JB, Tillet Y, Coudert AC, Oberli F, Preshaw P, et al. Efficacy of a new oral lubricant solution in the management of psychotropic drug-induced xerostomia: a randomized controlled trial. J Clin Psychopharmacol. 2007;27(5):437–43.

Chapter 44
Sedation

Sedation is sometimes reported as fatigue by patients. Fatigue or sedation can be caused by many systemic illnesses. In psychiatric patients, it could be a potential side effect of medications or a consequence of insomnia from the underlying illness. Obstructive sleep apnea (OSA) is a frequently unrecognized cause of poor sleep and daytime sedation. As OSA is associated with serious cardiovascular comorbidities, patients reporting poor sleep should be screened. Asking about snoring and apneic breathing and assessing for risk factors of obesity and hypertension are sufficient for initial screening.

Psychotropic Medications and Sedation

Medications with antihistaminic properties generally are the agents most likely to cause sedation. Among antipsychotics, olanzapine, clozapine, quetiapine, chlorpromazine, and ziprasidone are sedating. Among mood stabilizers, carbamazepine and valproate are likely to cause sedation. Among antidepressants, mirtazapine is the most sedating followed by paroxetine.

Sedation is generally managed by adjusting timing of medication so all or most of the dosing occurs at bedtime. Dose reduction, if possible, will also help. Modafinil and stimulants may be considered to promote wakefulness but is generally not recommended unless other indications for these agents are present.

> *Obstructive sleep apnea should always be considered in someone with daytime sedation.*
>
> *Medications with antihistaminic properties cause sedation.*
>
> *Reducing dose and changing time of administration is generally sufficient to counter this side effect.*

© Springer International Publishing AG 2017

A. Annamalai, *Medical Management of Psychotropic Side Effects,*
DOI 10.1007/978-3-319-51026-2_44

Chapter 45
Priapism

Priapism is a prolonged, persistent, and often painful penile erection, not usually initiated by sexual activity. A common cause among adults is intracavernous drug therapy for erectile dysfunction. Medical conditions that can cause it include hematologic disorders (e.g., sickle cell disease, leukemias), perineal trauma, and medications (e.g., anticoagulants, some antihypertensives). Patients with priapism generally have significant pain.

Psychotropic Medications and Priapism

Psychotropic medications are rarely associated with priapism. The mechanism is thought to be alpha adrenergic blockage of receptors in the corpora cavernosa of the penis. Trazodone and phenothiazine antipsychotics are implicated in a majority of cases [1]. Many case reports exist for low-potency typical antipsychotics. Fewer case reports are recorded for high-potency typical antipsychotics and atypical antipsychotics. Prazosin, often used in psychiatric practice, can also cause priapism.

An episode of priapism usually occurs upon starting an offending medication, raising the dose, or introduction of an additional risk factor. Recreational substances including alcohol, cocaine, and cannabis are all risk factors.

Regardless of cause, it should be treated as a clinical emergency and evaluated immediately by a urologist. If not treated promptly (aspiration of corpora cavernosa or intracavernous injection with alpha agonist), it may cause permanent impotence. For patients on psychotropic medications that could cause priapism, medication should be stopped and if possible, an agent with lesser alpha-blocking properties should be used.

© Springer International Publishing AG 2017

285

A. Annamalai, *Medical Management of Psychotropic Side Effects*,
DOI 10.1007/978-3-319-51026-2_45

> ***Priapism is a persistent penile erection that is occasionally caused by psychotropic medications. Trazodone and phenothiazine antipsychotics are commonly implicated.***
>
> ***If priapism occurs on psychotropic medication in the absence of other etiologies, medication should be switched to one with a lesser potential for alpha-blocking properties.***

Reference

1. Compton MT, Miller AH. Priapism associated with conventional and atypical antipsychotic medications: a review. J Clin Psychiatry. 2001;62(5):362–6.

Chapter 46
Polycystic Ovarian Syndrome

Polycystic ovarian syndrome (PCOS) is a common endocrine disorder in women. It is related to ovarian androgen excess and manifests as hirsutism, irregular menstrual cycles, and ovarian cysts seen on an ultrasonogram. Two out of three features are required to make a diagnosis. Obesity is often associated with PCOS. Symptoms are usually seen from puberty.

The androgen excess in PCOS results from increased ovarian androgen secretion and reduced conversion to estrogen. PCOS is associated with insulin resistance and hyperinsulinemia. These women are at increased risk for infertility and metabolic syndrome and its cardiovascular complications.

Valproate and PCOS

PCOS has been observed at a higher incidence in patients on valproate. It was initially observed in people on treatment for seizure disorder and it was uncertain whether valproate or the underlying seizure disorder predisposed to PCOS. PCOS was subsequently seen in patients being treated for bipolar disorder and was more frequent in those on valproate than other mood stabilizers [1]. It occurred within a year of treatment initiation. The mechanism is thought to be both from gamma aminobutyric acid (GABA)-mediated transmission to the hypothalamus and peripheral effect on estrogen and progesterone [2].

PCOS remits in most, but not all, patients who stop valproate even when weight gain from valproate persists [3]. The resolution of symptoms occurs within several months of stopping medication.

Valproate is not contraindicated in women with preexisting PCOS. If patients treated with valproate complain of new onset menstrual irregularity or increased hair growth, valproate-induced PCOS should be considered as a potential cause.

© Springer International Publishing AG 2017
A. Annamalai, *Medical Management of Psychotropic Side Effects*,
DOI 10.1007/978-3-319-51026-2_46

Patients who gain weight on valproate should be assessed for development of reproductive symptoms. Other causes of weight gain or menstrual irregularities (e.g., menopause, hyperprolactinemia) should also be considered.

If PCOS symptoms develop during treatment with valproate, stopping the medication should be considered, especially if the woman wishes to retain fertility. Patients can be referred to reproductive medicine or endocrinology for a definitive diagnosis before valproate is stopped or if symptoms persist after stopping valproate.

> ***PCOS is associated with valproate use though the causal role is not fully established. Stopping valproate usually causes remission of PCOS symptoms. A reproductive medicine or endocrinology consult is useful both for definitive diagnosis and treatment.***

References

1. Joffe H, Cohen LS, Suppes T, McLaughlin WL, Lavori P, Adams JM, et al. Valproate is associated with newonset oligoamenorrhea with hyperandrogenism in women with bipolar disorder. Biol Psychiatry. 2006;59(11):1078–86.
2. McIntyre RS, Mancini DA, McCann S, Srinivasan J, Kennedy SH. Valproate, bipolar disorder and polycystic ovarian syndrome. Bipolar Disord. 2003;5(1):28–35.
3. Joffe H, Cohen LS, Suppes T, Hwang CH, Molay F, Adams JM, et al. Longitudinal follow-up of reproductive and metabolic features of valproate-associated polycystic ovarian syndrome features: a preliminary report. Biol Psychiatry. 2006;60(12):1378–81.

Chapter 47
Osteoporosis

Osteoporosis is a condition of low bone mass. The prevalence increases with age and postmenopausal status in women. In both men and women, low physical activity, decreased calcium and vitamin D intake, cigarette smoking, and alcohol consumption are all risk factors. It can occur secondarily due to systemic illnesses. The main clinical impact of osteoporosis is increased risk for fractures.

Psychotropic Medications and Osteoporosis

Risk of osteoporosis appears to be increased in patients on selective serotonergic reuptake inhibitors (SSRIs). The risk starts in the first few months of treatment and diminishes about a year after stopping the medication. Tricyclic antidepressants (TCAs) also increase the risk [1]. The mechanism is thought to be via serotonergic receptors in bone cells. Anticonvulsant medications also affect bone density by effects on vitamin D, parathyroid hormone, and calcitonin metabolism. Antipsychotics affect bone density by elevating prolactin levels.

Psychiatric disorders, notably depression, inherently carry a risk of reduced bone density. The extent of risk attributable to psychotropic medications alone is still not clearly defined. There are no current guidelines on managing osteoporosis risk in patients on SSRIs or other psychotropic medications.

There is an increased risk of osteoporosis observed with many psychotropic medications but evidence is unclear on extent of risk and clinical impact.

© Springer International Publishing AG 2017   289
A. Annamalai, *Medical Management of Psychotropic Side Effects*,
DOI 10.1007/978-3-319-51026-2_47

Reference

1. Rizzoli R, Cooper C, Reginster JY, et al. Antidepressant medications and osteoporosis. Bone. 2012;51(3):606–13.

Chapter 48
Drug-Induced Lupus

Drug-induced lupus (DIL) is a syndrome with features similar to idiopathic systemic lupus erythematosus (SLE). The mechanism is not known and it may vary depending on the particular medication. It is not clear if DIL exacerbates symptoms in preexisting lupus, induces lupus in susceptible patients, or causes a distinct entity of DIL. Regardless of the pathway, the pathology is enhanced autoimmunity.

Common symptoms are fever, myalgias, rash, and arthralgias. Systemic organ involvement (renal, hematologic, central nervous system) is less common than with SLE. A cutaneous lupus can also be seen in which the skin eruptions are more widespread than in idiopathic cutaneous lupus. In DIL, autoantibodies (antinuclear antibodies and other lupus specific antibodies) are elevated as in idiopathic SLE.

Psychotropic Medications and Lupus

Psychotropic medications are rarely associated with lupus. There are case reports with carbamazepine, valproate, and lithium. The manifestations usually occur within a month of exposure. Stopping the offending medication appears to resolve symptoms and reverse lab abnormalities in weeks to months [1]. Presence of SLE is not a contraindication to using one of these agents but patients should be monitored for any worsening of lupus symptoms. If there is new onset or worsening lupus symptoms, medication should be switched to an alternative agent.

Mood stabilizers (valproate, carbamazepine, lamotrigine) are occasionally associated with drug-induced lupus.

© Springer International Publishing AG 2017

A. Annamalai, *Medical Management of Psychotropic Side Effects*,

DOI 10.1007/978-3-319-51026-2_48

Reference

1. Park-Matsumoto YC, Tazawa T. Valproate induced lupus-like syndrome. J Neurol Sci. 1996;143(1–2):185–6.

Chapter 49
Cataracts

Cataract is an opacity of the lens in the eye. It can cause blindness when the opacity is complete. It is a slowly occurring process with advancing age. In addition to age, cigarette smoking, alcohol consumption, sunlight exposure, and metabolic syndrome add to the risk.

Psychotropic Medications and Cataracts

Cataracts appear to occur at an increased frequency with typical antipsychotic medications, especially phenothiazines [1]. The risk is difficult to quantify as cataracts develop over time and drug-related cataracts cannot be distinguished from naturally occurring senile cataracts. There are occasional case reports of cataract formation with haloperidol. Quetiapine carries a manufacturer recommendation to perform routine eye examinations though a causal link is not established. There are no recommendations for managing cataract risk on antipsychotics except possibly for periodic eye examinations.

Phenothiazines appear to be associated with an increased frequency of cataract formation.

Reference

1. Shahzad S, Suleman MI, Shahab H, Mazour I, Kaur A, Rudzinskiy P, et al. Cataract occurrence with antipsychotic drugs. Psychosomatics. 2002;43(5):354–9.

© Springer International Publishing AG 2017   293
A. Annamalai, *Medical Management of Psychotropic Side Effects*,
DOI 10.1007/978-3-319-51026-2_49

Chapter 50
Nephrolithiasis

Kidney stones are solid particle formations in the urinary tract. They are not uncommon in the general population. Majority of stones are formed of calcium. They may be passed into the bladder and excreted in urine or lodged in the urinary tract causing irritation and obstruction. Kidney stones can cause severe pain and accompanying nausea. Patients may also present with hematuria or symptoms of a urinary tract infection.

Topiramate and Nephrolithiasis

Kidney stones can occasionally be seen with topiramate treatment. The prevalence of symptomatic nephrolithiasis on topiramate may be as high as 10% [1]. The mechanism is thought to be inhibition of renal carbonic anhydrase and renal tubular acidosis. The metabolic acidosis leads to formation of alkaline urine, reduced citrate, and increased calcium in the urine predisposing to calcium phosphate stones.

There is limited evidence to guide management of nephrolithiasis on topiramate treatment. If patient has a history of metabolic acidosis, chronic renal disease, or prior stone formation, topiramate can be avoided as a first-line agent. If stone formation occurs on topiramate treatment, medication should be stopped and patient referred for appropriate acute treatment of nephrolithiasis as well as preventive management.

Topiramate may cause kidney stones in up to 10% patients. In patients with a prior history of nephrolithiasis, topiramate may be avoided as a first-line agent.

© Springer International Publishing AG 2017
A. Annamalai, *Medical Management of Psychotropic Side Effects*,
DOI 10.1007/978-3-319-51026-2_50

Reference

1. Maalouf NM, Langston JP, Van Ness PC, Moe OW, Sakhaee K. Nephrolithiasis in topiramate users. Urol Res. 2011;39(4):303–7.

Index

A

Abdominal pain, 25, 148, 156, 157, 160, 161
Abnormal involuntary movements (AIMS)
    scale, 238
Absolute neutrophil count (ANC), 177, 178,
    180–183
Acetylcholine, 271
Acute confusional state, 271
Acute hyperglycemia, 272, 274
    clinical features, 25
    overview, 27–29
    psychotropic medications, 24
Acute hypertriglyceridemia, 42
Acute liver failure, 149
Acute pancreatitis, 155
Agranulocytosis, 9, 176–179, 181, 182
Akathisia, 171, 221, 222, 235, 236, 239–240
Albumin creatinine ratio (ACR), 123
Alcohol use, 42, 50, 135, 152, 155, 189
Alpha adrenergic blockade, 48, 139
Alpha-blocking properties, 285
Alpha-glucosidase inhibitors, 29
Altered mental status
    etiologies of delirium, 271–272
    pathology, 271
Amantadine, 232, 234, 239, 240
American College of Cardiology (ACC),
    41, 43
American Heart Association (AHA), 41, 43
Amiloride, 112
Amylase, 157, 158
Anemia, 176, 193, 197, 198
    clinical features, 194
    definition, 193
    diagnosis, 195

etiology, 194, 195
management, 195
pathology, 193
psychotropic medications, 194
Angiotensin receptor blockers (ARBs), 37
Angiotensin-converting enzyme inhibitors
    (ACEIs), 37
Anorexia, 60, 104, 150
Anticholinergic(s), 137–139, 160, 239, 276
Anticholinergic agent, 117, 166, 236–238, 240
Anticholinergic delirium, 252, 272, 273
Anticholinergic medications, 135, 167,
    238–240, 272
Antidepressants, 4, 7, 8, 10, 11, 16, 32, 40,
    48, 74, 75, 86, 87, 95, 130, 131,
    133–135, 138, 139, 147–149,
    156, 160, 170, 176, 179, 211,
    226, 232, 251, 264, 265, 272,
    273, 276, 283, 289
Antidiuretic hormone (ADH), 115, 118
Antihistaminic properties, 283
Antipsychotics, 4, 6–8, 11, 16, 24, 26, 40, 48,
    54, 74, 87, 89, 116, 148, 149, 156,
    157, 160, 165, 179, 180, 226, 235,
    265, 283
Aripiprazole, 138, 141, 232, 236
Arthralgias, 291
Athetosis, 222
Atrioventricular (AV) block
    clinical features, 68–69
    diagnosis, 69
    etiology, 67
    management, 69–71
    pathology, 67
    psychotropic medications, 68

A. Annamalai, *Medical Management of Psychotropic Side Effects*,
DOI 10.1007/978-3-319-51026-2

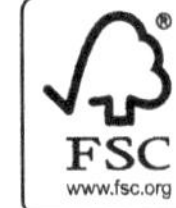

If you have any concerns about our products,
you can contact us on
ProductSafety@springernature.com

In case Publisher is established outside the EU,
the EU authorized representative is:
Springer Nature Customer Service Center GmbH
Europaplatz 3, 69115 Heidelberg, Germany

Printed by Libri Plureos GmbH
in Hamburg, Germany